CW00530848

A PROPHET IN HIS OWN COUNTRY

By the same author

'*Unrecognised by the World at Large*'
A biography of Dr Henry Parsey MD, the first Physician to the
Warwick County Asylum

A PROPHET IN HIS OWN COUNTRY

*

A biography of
Henry Lilley Smith (1788–1859)
Member of the Royal College of Surgeons of London

'Surgeon Oculist & Aurist' of Southam, Warwickshire;
founder of its Infirmary for the Treatment of Diseases of the Eye &
Ear in 1818, and who established the first Provident Dispensary
'in the Kingdom' in 1823

*

ALASTAIR ROBSON

'A prophet is not without honour save in his own country'

Copyright © 2023 Alastair Robson

The moral right of the author has been asserted.

Apart from any fair dealing for the purposes of research or private study,
or criticism or review, as permitted under the Copyright, Designs and Patents
Act 1988, this publication may only be reproduced, stored or transmitted, in
any form or by any means, with the prior permission in writing of the
publishers, or in the case of reprographic reproduction in accordance with
the terms of licences issued by the Copyright Licensing Agency. Enquiries
concerning reproduction outside those terms should be sent to the publishers.

Matador
Unit E2 Airfield Business Park,
Harrison Road, Market Harborough,
Leicestershire. LE16 7UL
Tel: 0116 2792299
Email: books@troubador.co.uk
Web: www.troubador.co.uk/matador
Twitter: @matadorbooks

ISBN 978 1803134 895

British Library Cataloguing in Publication Data.
A catalogue record for this book is available from the British Library.

Printed and bound in Great Britain by 4edge Limited
Typeset in 11pt Minion Pro by Troubador Publishing Ltd, Leicester, UK

Matador is an imprint of Troubador Publishing Ltd

To Ann, Andrew and Helen

CONTENTS

List of Illustrations

1. Henry Lilley Smith in later life: from an old photograph.
2. The Eye & Ear Infirmary today.
3. The Henry Lilley Smith Memorial.
4. Market Hill in 1804.
5. St James's Church, Southam c.1871.
6. All Saints Church, Ladbroke.
7. 'A Vestry Dinner' – a cartoon by Isaac Cruikshank (1795).
8. 'A Surgical Operation to Remove a Malignant Tumour from a Man's Left Breast and Armpit in a Dublin Drawing Room' (1817).
9. 'The Country Infirmary' – a cartoon by Charles Williams (1813).
10. The surgical operation of 'couching' a cataract of the eye.
11. The Eye & Ear Infirmary c.1850.
12. Southam's ancient Holy Well.
13. The Dispensary and the Infirmary c.1823.
14. St Peter's Church, Dorsington c.1871.
15. Clapham Dispensary today.

SOURCE OF ILLUSTRATIONS: 1, 5, 9 courtesy of Wellcome Collection (Attribution 4.0 International [CC BY 4.0]; 2, 3, 6, 12 author's photographs; 4, 5, 13 illustrations by Sophia Smith for William Lilley Smith's History of Southam; 11 courtesy of Southam Heritage Collection; 7 courtesy of Chris Beetles Gallery, St James's, London; 10 courtesy of Unite for Sight; 14 pen and ink drawing by Sophia Smith – original in author's possession; courtesy of 'Clapham through Time' (image edit: Christina Bonnet; original image courtesy of Google Maps).

Author's Note

This is an informal study of Henry Lilley Smith; I have therefore omitted references for every quotation given, but I have included a comprehensive bibliography.

However, where I felt items of information did not sit well with the flow of the text, I have added footnotes – be they either to inform, or merely amuse, the reader.

Acknowledgements

I am indebted to Linda Doyle, of Southam's Heritage Collection, who suggested that a biography of Henry Lilley Smith should accompany the Heritage Collection's forthcoming exhibition in 2023 for the bicentenary of his provident dispensary on Warwick Road – 'the first in the Kingdom' – and who made available to me much background material from the Collection.

Despite the increased rigours of NHS medical practice during the last couple of years, Professor Gary Misson FRCS, FRCOphth and Mr David Phillips FRCS found time to advise me on aspects of surgery of the eye and ear in the nineteenth century; Dr John Wilmot MRCGP provided much additional information about Warwickshire's charitable dispensaries.

Primary sources were also consulted in the Warwick County Record Office, the National Archives at Kew, and the library of the National Army Museum in Chelsea.

Any author writing about Henry Lilley Smith is especially indebted to Simon Wheeler's 1996 MA thesis for Warwick University entitled 'Henry Lilley Smith (1788–1859): surgeon, philanthropist and originator of provident dispensaries: a study of the career, ideas and achievements of a nineteenth-century country doctor' – the first serious study of his life and practice.

It has been said elsewhere that writing books is a pastime that requires heroic tolerance by the rest of the family – very grateful thanks are due therefore to my wife, Ann, for enthusiastically accompanying me on visits to churches, tombs, and other local buildings of interest, and for her forbearance during the writing of this book.

In Samuel Beckett's opinion, 'the most desirable biography should include the straws, flotsam, etc.; names, dates, births and deaths...' I have tried to follow his advice.

A.M.R.
Southam, Warwickshire
March 2022

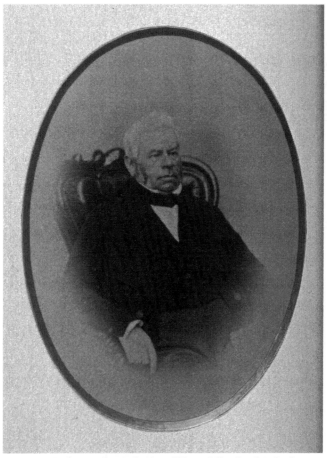

Illustration 1: A photomechanical print of Henry Lilley Smith in his later years, by J E Duggins.

Introduction

A visitor to Southam today, entering the town by car via the Warwick Road, is very likely to overlook the modest memorial in front of an imposing building on the left-hand side of the road, just before it takes the traveller over the bridge across the River Stowe, and up the rise to Market Hill.

The building itself, now Grade II listed, is of 'rendered brick with pilasters to front; 8-window range of pointed-arch casements with Gothick glazing bars to first and second storeys; nineteenth-century sashes to ground floor with canted bays'. Now a wedding venue, known as 'Warwick House', but for many years previously the 'Stoneythorpe Hotel', it had been opened in 1818 as an 'Infirmary for the Curing of Diseases of the Eye and Ear' by Henry Lilley Smith, Member of the Royal College of Surgeons of London, whose entire medical career was spent in Southam as a 'surgeon oculist and aurist', or specialist in diseases of the eye and ear.

If the traveller is curious enough to stop to inspect the memorial more closely, what is to be found?

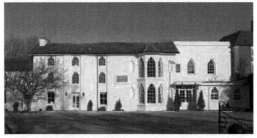

Illustration 2: The Eye & Ear Infirmary today (now known as 'Warwick House').

Set back a little from the road, a large stone urn stands upon a four-sided limestone column, bearing inscriptions on each side, mounted on a large granite plinth and enclosed by iron railings.

What does the inscription on the side facing the road say?

THIS STONE
MARKS THE SITE OF THE
DISPENSARY COTTAGE
used for the purposes of the
first self-supporting
PROVIDENT DISPENSARY
IN THE KINGDOM
established here by
Mr H. L. SMITH
in the year 1823
upon the plan afterwards
so successfully adopted at
COVENTRY, NORTHAMPTON
AND MANY OTHER PLACES

*

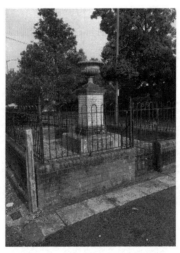

Illustration 3: Memorial to Henry Lilley Smith facing onto Warwick Road.

This book is a study of the life of 'Mr H. L. Smith' (as he is so commemorated), an eye and ear surgeon in rural nineteenth-century Warwickshire, and his 'Infirmary for the Treatment of Diseases of the Eye and Ear' and 'Provident Dispensary – for the better provision of medical care for the labouring classes and their families' – which by the end of the century had been copied throughout the country, and then adopted by Lloyd George's National Insurance Act of 1911 as national policy for health care.

1

EARLY LIFE

Henry Lilley Smith was Southam born and bred.[1] His date of birth is not recorded but he was baptised on 25th March 1788, in St James's Church, Southam, where his father, William Lilley Smith, had been married by William Bellamy, curate, to Sophia Chambers on 3rd April the previous year: the marriage was witnessed by Sophia's father Henry Chambers and William Basse, the Parish Clerk.

At the time of Henry's baptism his father William (also born in Southam, in 1766) was described as a 'grocer'. Henry's mother, Sophia Chambers, was likewise Southam born and bred, and she was also baptised in St James's, on 8th June 1763. Henry's father lived until 1844, aged eighty-four, and his mother died in 1861 at the grand age of ninety-eight. Both parents were buried in the family tomb, regrettably now fallen into disrepair, in the churchyard of St James' Church.

Henry's paternal grandfather, Lilley Smith, had been born in Coventry in 1725; his wife's name was Susanna. Later in life he lived in Warwick, where he died on 2nd April 1807; he had property in Coventry and was described in the burial register of

---

1   For an introduction to the small Warwickshire market town of Southam (pop. c.1,000 in 1788), see 'Chapter 3 – Return to Southam'.

St Mary's Church, Warwick, as a 'gentleman alderman, formerly of Coventry', although he had described himself as 'oilman' in his will of 1802.

Henry's maternal grandfather, Henry Chambers, was also Southam born: his wife Hannah's family, the Pearsons, were property owners in Bishop's Itchington, some four miles distant. He died in 1823 and was buried in the family tomb. He was described as a 'mercer' and the Chambers family were also people of property – owning a substantial farmhouse and three acres of land in Napton – and were Southam's local drapers for many years, occupying one of the houses on the high street opposite Market Hill.

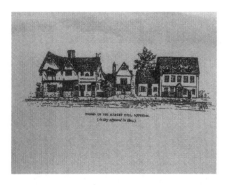

Illustration 4: Market Hill, Southam in 1804 (The Chambers family probably lived in one of these houses) – drawing by Sophia Smith.

William was described in documents as a grocer until at least 1809, but his social position in the town advanced in later years: in 1803 William was one of only eight Southam residents on the Jury List,[2] but by 1817 he was described as 'Gentleman' on the much-expanded Jury List of twenty-three Southam residents and by 1835 he was listed as 'Esq.' in the Warwickshire Directory of Southam's 'Nobility, Gentry and Clergy', his name immediately following the entry for 'Sir Francis Shuckburgh, Bart.'

2   Eligibility for jury service required the juror to be male and a freeholder of property: juries were therefore substantial householders in the main, and invariably members of the 'middling sort', such as farmers, tradesmen or other craftsmen.

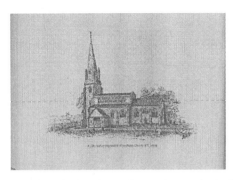

Illustration 5: St James's Church, Southam – drawing by Sophia Smith.

Henry Lilley Smith was an only child, and details of his early years and schooling are sparse: he appears to have commenced schooling in Southam at a surprisingly early age, according to a letter written to his mother by her father, Henry Chambers, Henry's grandfather, dated 'Southam, 13th November 1790':

> 'My dear Sophia,
> … your dear boy had a bad cold about a week ago and was poorly for two or three nights but made no complaint by day and went daily to school and thank God he is now quite well… I believe he is as good and happy a child as any in this world of his age – he is everything you could wish him to be…'

Fulsome, if grandfatherly, praise indeed; but then, to be informed of illness in one's child needs rapid reassurance that all is now well, especially if he has been left in the care of his grandparents. But why was that?

From the few letters from Henry Chambers to his daughter preserved in the County Record Office, it seems that Henry's parents went to live in Woodbridge, Suffolk, (population c.5,000) in October 1790, where William continued in trade as a grocer, but with a struggle; at one stage they required financial support from both sets of parents, according to the correspondence which is not particularly forthcoming as to why – there is some suggestion that trade was

3

poor, presumably due to the price of corn rising steadily from crop failures in the early 1790s, and it was presumably this which forced them to return to Southam in July 1791, initially to lodge with Sophia's parents. The reasons for them deciding to leave Henry with his maternal grandparents during this period is not known.

The most interesting fact that emerges from this letter is that Henry appears to be going to school aged two and a half years. He would have been too young to enter the charity school that existed in Southam, so presumably this was a local 'dame school', which were often to be found in rural areas, invariably run by women from their homes whilst they carried on with their domestic duties, and for the most part provided child care to the very young. But, in their defence, the observation was made in 1835 that 'Dame schools have become almost universal; and defective as they may be in their plans of instruction, many a child has reason to look back upon scenes of his earliest days with gratitude to God for the benefits he received in those humble and imperfectly-managed nurseries.'

According to the medical historian Irvine Loudon:

> 'The typical surgeon or surgeon-apothecary was a grammar school boy, and his success at school was measured in terms of the extent of his reading in the classics. He left school between the ages of twelve and fifteen with at least some knowledge of Latin and often a smattering of Greek. Then he became an apprentice.'[3]

That being the case, one might assume that Henry would have gone on to attend one of the local grammar schools, but there is no record of his being enrolled as a pupil at Warwick School, Rugby School, King Henry VIII School, Coventry, or King Edward VI School, Stratford-upon-Avon – all of which were then 'free grammar schools' – so presumably he was educated in Southam at the charity school, which had been established in the 1760s.

---

3   See bibliography.

A 'Deed of Bargain and Sale of an Estate in Southam' in the Record Office, dated 6th April 1762, states that Lord Craven, Sir Charles Skipwith, and others 'were desirous to found a charity school on lands in the Parish of Southam for the children of the poor inhabitants of the town, for instructing them in the principles of the Church of England and in reading and saying their catechisms and spinning, working of plain work and other proper and useful learning for poor children and for the buying of books for their improvement and for the supplying of a fit schoolmaster or schoolmistress or both... who shall be at liberty to take any other scholars to the said school beside the said poor children of the Parish of Southam.'

A directory of residents of Southam for 1793–1798 lists a 'William Alport, schoolteacher': in which case, the charity school was certainly active in Henry Lilley Smith's school years, and although he was hardly a child of 'poor inhabitants' – his family were property owners, after all – the school had discretion to accept other children who showed aptitude. He, presumably, was one of those.

Schooling provision in the town in later years improved considerably when the National School building in School Street opened in 1816: built 'in the gothic style', with its central house providing accommodation for the schoolteacher and his family and schoolrooms for sixty boys and girls, with distinctly separate entrances at each end, it is now a pre-school nursery.[4]

In an 1828 directory, as well as the National School, there was an 'Academy' run by a Catherine Harris which accepted 'ladies for day and boarding' – affordable only by a minority of families, one suspects.

By 1842, with the expansion of the town, five private schools in Southam were listed, including a second 'Academy for boarding and day pupils', run by a Revd William Williams, but further information regarding Henry's school years is lacking.

---

4   National Schools were founded in 1811 'to provide elementary education to poor children', again 'in accordance with the Church of England'. Compulsory education from the ages of five to twelve would not be established in England until 1870.

2

APPRENTICESHIP

Henry's charity school education plainly gave him a decent academic grounding, for in 1804 at the age of sixteen he was indentured as an apprentice to Mr Thomas Nicholls Adams MRCS, LSA, 'Surgeon and Apothecary', of Park Street, Walsall: the five-year apprenticeship would have cost his parents about £120 in total, including Henry's board and lodging, but 'excluding clothes'.

In 1804, Walsall was a flourishing Staffordshire town with a racecourse, manufacturing mainly 'horse furniture' and other iron, brass and leather wares applicable to carriages etc., with a population of about 10,400 (by the end of the century its population would be 86,400). Henry would have been kept well occupied in assisting Mr Adams in the day-to-day running of the medical practice of a busy single-handed 'surgeon-apothecary'.

His maternal grandfather continued to take a close interest in his only grandchild and his education over the years; Henry appears to have been an amiable child, as far as available reports go. A letter to his daughter Sophia, Henry's mother, written on 2nd December 1790, after Henry's paternal grandparents, Lilley and Susanna Smith, had been staying with Henry Chambers, survives in the sparse correspondence from the Woodbridge years: 'I did many things to make them comfortable and I did not labour in vain. They were very fond of your dear boy. Indeed it is hardly possible not to be, for he is a dear good child… and I was pleased [I was] not jealous of his love to them.'

In a letter dated 29th September 1804, soon after Henry had arrived in Walsall, Henry Chambers appears to have been somewhat alarmed by an unknown comment Henry must have said or written to him, which provoked the response: 'Southam is better than the South of France – and much safer.' One can only surmise.

In June 1805 he wrote again, enclosing 'a small bill' – this was invariably a £10 banknote, then quite a substantial sum indeed.[5] In February 1806 he wrote and commented, enigmatically: 'You will sometimes know what a dangerous age 17 is' – presumably in response to further confidences between grandson and grandfather (now lost) – about the usual distractions at that age, no doubt?

In January 1808 he writes again, enclosing another £10 banknote, 'for fear you should think yourself going poor.' Very indulgent, but what was Henry up to? He seems to be indulging in profligate spending (in Walsall?) – although this appears a touch out of character – as if he were in the South of France, perhaps?

Henry remained with Mr Adams for four years and seems to have applied himself to his studies diligently, for in October 1808, he was accepted by 'The United Hospitals of Guy and St Thomas' in London as a 'surgical dresser' for six months, probably with the intention of presenting himself for examination at the Royal College of Surgeons the following May.

An apprenticeship to a provincial 'surgeon and apothecary', whilst providing good experience of the practicalities of day-to-day general medical practice – and much mundane activity besides, such as bottle washing, sweeping the surgery, running errands

---

5   £10 in 1800 would have had the purchasing power of almost £500 today.

and grooming the horse(s) – was sufficient perhaps for obtaining the apothecary's licence by examination from Apothecaries Hall in London (LSA),[6] but a surgical career would require broader experience, obtained only by encountering patients on the wards and in the outpatients departments of a busy hospital; and it was an essential requirement of the Royal College of Surgeons that all candidates for the diploma of Membership of the College had to 'walk the wards' and 'attend a course of instruction in a hospital of more than 100 beds' – in London, Edinburgh, Aberdeen or Dublin – 'for a minimum of six months' before taking the exam. Students gravitated in the main towards the London hospitals, especially 'The United Borough Hospitals of Guy and St Thomas' in Southwark, where there was an established medical school which provided the necessary courses of instruction in anatomy, surgery, midwifery, medicine and chemistry. The fee for such a course of lectures was £70 (a substantial fee indeed, when a five-year apprenticeship cost £120).

At Guy's, each surgeon had four student dressers – for a further fee – who, by rotation, were resident in the hospital for a week at a time, who assisted at operations and attended to the day-to-day needs of the patients whilst in the wards. Quite an arduous task, for surgical wounds in those days invariably became infected, and would require frequent dressing and re-dressing. Henry was fortunate to have been made a dresser to Mr Astley Cooper, who was a Lecturer in Surgery and Anatomy at Guy's, and apparently an outstanding teacher and surgeon, whose lectures and ward rounds were crowded 'to overflowing' with students.[7]

---

6   LSA: Licence of the Society of Apothecaries, often referred to – not entirely in jest – as 'the licence to kill', allowed the holder to legally make and dispense medication. In 1815 it became a compulsory qualification for practice as a doctor, in an attempt to identify and reduce 'quackery' (unqualified, and often expensive, practitioners).

7   Sir Astley Cooper (1768–1841): Surgeon at Guy's Hospital from 1810. Described as 'indefatigable'. He removed a cyst from the scalp of King George IV in 1817 and was rewarded with a knighthood.

Dressers also attended to the various conditions seen in the outpatient department – acute infections, some for lancing, more dressings, dental extractions, setting broken limbs and helping to deal with the many injuries – some severe – involving horses and carriages. Arduous perhaps, but for a student a coveted position of some responsibility.

A contemporary of Henry's at Guy's, William Dent, wrote in a letter of 5th December 1808, to his mother: 'We have a great deal of practice in the hospitals, and accidents are continually brought in; we have the opportunity of seeing them all. Seldom a day but something remarkable happens.'

During some of his time at Guy's, Henry lodged at the house of James Durie MRCS, a surgeon, in Great Suffolk Street, just off Borough High Street, at the southern end of London Bridge and close to the hospital. Whether he was also tutored by him, we don't know. Possibly.

William Dent lodged at 4 Thomas's Tents, also just a few doors from Guy's Hospital, with two other medical students; their days were occupied with lectures and the anatomy room. They appear to have been studious (for the most part), 'writing out the lectures that we hear till 12 or one o'clock every night', according to William.

Borough, south of the river, was a notorious and squalid area of London; 'a beastly place in dirt, turnings and windings' was John Keats' opinion, in a letter written when he was himself lodging in Thomas's Street in 1815–1817, when he too was a surgical dresser at Guy's. (John Keats, allegedly, 'dressed à la Byron' and developed 'a taste for claret, snuff and cigars' whilst at Guy's. In spite of having also 'learned to play billiards and whist', and attending 'boxing matches, cockfights and bear-baitings', it was not all play and no work, however, for he was awarded the diploma from Apothecaries' Hall [LSA] in 1816. London has always had its temptations and medical students have long had a reputation for studying hard and playing hard, but I sense Henry

Lilley Smith would have disapproved of such behaviour most strongly – as we shall discover later.

Ever the penniless medical student, Dent wrote home in the same letter of December 1808:

'Everything is excessively dear: three of us pay 18s. week for lodgings and we find ourselves of everything we want, when on average it costs us 25s. week but, however, I can tell you I am really as careful as I can possibly be.'

He, like every other medical student from time immemorial, regularly requested money from home, and the method of sending it which he suggested to his parents seems to have been fairly standard practice in those days:

'If you will send me a note in your next letter which you may do with great safety, by tearing it in two and sending each half in separate letters, but don't send both letters on the same day. This is the way two young men have received money from home and it came very safe.'

Henry still received letters in London from his grandfather, too; the last of the small collection which has survived was written on 11th January 1809 and addressed to Henry at Great Suffolk Street: 'I have enclosed another £10 bill [untorn], a gift to buy Cowper's Poems (2 vols @ 16s.).': 'rather than drink', one can almost read between the lines.[8]

He then goes on to add 'hands, eyes, memory, all failing...' (but, in fact, Henry Chambers lived until he was aged ninety-two and managed to see his grandson qualified and established in practice in Southam).

---

8   William Cowper (1731–1800): one of the most popular poets of his time, he wrote of life in the English countryside and also the hymn which begins 'God moves in a mysterious way/His wonders to perform'.

Instruction at Guy's was as much practical as academic – more from William Dent:

'I am attending midwifery and I have had one labour. I managed all tolerably well, and the woman is doing famously now. I expect to have another shortly, but the worst of it is, we have to give them 5 shillings and find them with medicines until they are quite well.'

Henry must have done much the same – evidence of having attended an approved course of midwifery lectures (and they had been given at Guy's since before the end of the eighteenth century) was a pre-requisite for entry to the MRCS examination, although it was not a subject the College of Surgeons examined candidates on. Midwifery was a substantial burden for any country doctor; we know that Henry, when Parish Surgeon, attended one delivery and one miscarriage between January and April 1815, which he itemised in the account he submitted to the Overseer [see Appendix 2a]. No doubt there were other occasions, but evidence is lacking.

To return to Guy's, Henry, like Dent, continued 'walking the wards' until about February 1809. Some months later his father sent him a letter, addressed to 'Mr Henry Lilley Smith, Assistant Surgeon, Colchester Barracks'. Colchester? What was he doing there?

Another letter home from William Dent, written on 17th February 1809, reveals all:

'Mr Astley Cooper, the surgeon and Lecturer at St Thomas's, has received a letter from Mr Knight, Inspector of Hospitals, desiring all the students that possibly can leave town for to go to different districts to attend and dress the sick and wounded soldiers that have arrived from Spain for the wounded are so numerous and the Assistant Surgeons so scarce that the poor men are actually lost for want of surgical aid. Mr Cooper hoped that every young man that could go, would, for he looked upon it both as humanity and as a duty to do so in such an emergency. He said that they would have practice which it was impossible they could at present in London and as it would be only of a temporary nature not exceeding a month or six weeks, he trusted it would not interrupt our studies… I am going to Colchester, I and seven others [one of whom being Henry Lilley Smith] set out tomorrow morning. I beg your pardon for not asking your leave before I went but as it is on such urgent business, I hope you will be led to excuse me and that my conduct will meet with the approbation of yourself and all my friends. I assure you that if I thought I would not have benefitted from it I would never have attempted such a thing. We have our expenses found both there and back and £7 a month.'

The sudden influx of casualties to England was caused by the evacuation of the British Army from Spain after the disastrous Battle of Corunna on 16th January 1809.

When Henry Lilley Smith's obituarist in the *British Medical Journal* wrote 'he apparently served under Sir John Moore at Corunna', there is little supporting evidence – he was still in London, lodging in the house of Mr Durie, and involved with his medical studies at the time of the battle – he had received a letter from his grandfather dated 11th January 1809, after all, addressed to Great Suffolk Street. He was to be much involved in the medical care of the injured from the battle, though, once the soldiers had been repatriated from Spain in some disarray; 'every ship had orders to make for the first port in England they could'.

More than 6,000 men were classified as sick or injured on their arrival in England. And no wonder; the troops had had to endure a forced march of over 250 miles in mountainous country in the winter of 1808–1809 before the army managed to reach Corunna for the battle, and sickness among the troops in the Peninsular campaign was always a greater problem than casualties.

Dent's first letter from Colchester on 5th March 1809 sets the scene:

'I was very much surprised to find such a number of men sick as there is. There are only five Assistants at this place. [Assistant Surgeons were given the army rank of Subaltern, which gave them access to the Officers' Mess.] Each one is placed under a separate surgeon. I am placed under a very nice man of the name of Hill who is a surgeon to the 1st Battalion of the 4th Regiment[9] which is come from Spain and in that Regiment alone there is 197 men sick and wounded in the Hospital and half that number I have taken care of myself.'

But it was not all doom and gloom; he continues, appreciatively:

'I am very glad I came here for besides attending to the sick and wounded we have the privilege of dissecting those who die and in London we could not get a dead body under 3 gns.'

The duties at Colchester were arduous; Dent again:

'There are several regiments in this garrison that are very sickly indeed. Both battalions of the 43rd [10] and 76th [11] have a great number ill and several have died and they continue to take a good many into hospital every day. Every evening at about dusk a string of from eight to ten fine fellows are carried to their graves. The deaths are so

---

9   Since 1959, the 'King's Own Royal Border Regiment'.

10   Since 1968, the 'Royal Green Jackets'.

11   Since 1881, the 'Duke of Wellington's Regiment'.

numerous that a corporal and eight men only attended each funeral.'

Henry and William's pay as temporary Assistant Surgeons was £7 per month; rooming at Colchester Barracks cost 5s./week – furnished with bed, chest of drawers, mirror, carpet and washstand. Henry would have had a servant 'out of the ranks' to wait on him for 2s./week and, as a Subaltern, would mess with the other Officers of the Regiment (breakfast 1s. 0d., dinner 2s. 6d., supper 9d.) i.e. £2 5s. 0d. per month in total – excluding his mess bill (if any); a necessary expenditure, and usually considered to be quite expensive. It could have been worse. Regular Assistant Surgeons were paid 6s. 6d./day [£15/month]. On campaign, Regimental Surgeons in both infantry and cavalry regiments – but not Assistant Surgeons – were required to provide themselves with a horse (or two) at their own expense, but were given a daily 'forage allowance' to feed it. Dent and Henry were let off lightly.

A long letter from Henry's father, dated 19th May 1809, sent to Henry at Colchester, is quoted verbatim, as follows:

'Your mother and I are much concerned at your going but I suppose we must give consent [although Henry had turned 21 in March that year] as you seem so very desirous to go God protect you and I hope you will be careful of yourself and let us hear immediately from you if your mind is fully made up to go. You must come to Southam to take farewell.

Your mother thinks you see things in too favourable a light. She says the French are in possession of Italy and she thinks they will conquer Portugal as they have been successful. Your mother's chest trembles so much she is not able to write a line – setting aside our affection for you, think were his propriety would be to go to those that he has no regard for [sic]. We know the time would hang

14

heavy on your hands at Southam, but if you would get a situation to pass a few months at, you would then be within 2-3 days call if anything should happen to your grandfather or ourselves. You must excuse what I write as I have to know what I do write. Your grandpa is 82 though he wishes not to be thought above 78. If you are determined upon joining you will always have our blessing and good wishes. It will be impossible for us to come to you as we have 100 Irish soldiers come here to stay 2 or 3 months. The officers wish much to come to our house but we can't accommodate them; they give the soldiers a very bad character for every kind of mischief…[12]

Your grandpa and mother join with me in best wishes.
Believe me to be
Your affectionate father
W L Smith
PS If you get a situation will [you] endeavour to spare your mother to come to see you.'

So, it appears he was intending to join Wellington in the Peninsular War – presumably as an Assistant Surgeon in the Army Medical Service. Poor parents: by now, they had expected him to have qualified, but instead, here he was, diverted from his academic studies, and planning to join the army; no wonder they were 'concerned', and rightly so. But, in any event, this didn't happen – no doubt much to their relief.

Dent's absence from his studies lasted longer than the anticipated four to six weeks – he did not leave Colchester until September. It is probable that Henry's movements mirrored William's; if so, then they had both returned to their studies in London by the autumn of 1809: Astley Cooper's prediction of 'four to six weeks absence' from

---

12   Possibly from the 83rd (County of Dublin) Regiment of Foot – later the 'Royal Irish Rifles' – who were in England at that time, awaiting embarkation for Spain, where they fought at the Battle of Talavera on 27th/28th July 1809.

Guy's had turned out to be more than eight months. Henry would often refer to this period of his life in future years by saying, 'I was, for a short time in my career, attached to the Army' – 'attached' rather than 'commissioned' is probably correct; but he is forgiven – we have all inflated our CVs at some time or another...

Henry may have returned from Colchester to James Durie's house in Great Suffolk Street, but this is uncertain. However, January 1810 found William in new lodgings near St Thomas's; 'victuals, coals, candles, washing and everything included for 2gns/week'. Expenditure included 'a course of dissections for 5 gns, a body for 3 gns and a case of dissecting instruments for £2'.

The study of surgery requires the minutest familiarity with the anatomy of the human body; repeated dissection is the key to such an understanding. Here is a description of the anatomy room in the time of Sir Astley Cooper:

> 'Bodies were laid out on the ten or twelve dissection tables in the room, in various stages of decay depending on the swiftness with which they were removed from the churchyard after burial and the success, or otherwise, of the process of pickling in alcohol.'

The 'bodies' that Henry and William worked on were almost certainly procured for the Anatomy School at Guy's by Astley Cooper himself, who surreptitiously obtained them from the 'resurrection men' – the body-snatchers, who removed corpses from newly buried coffins at night and transferred them to anatomy schools – for a fee. The brisk (but, of course, quite illegal) trade was overlooked by the hospital authorities and the police.

Henry's mother's uncle, George Pearson, had stipulated in his will of 1792 that he and his wife 'be buried with a neat monument in plain marble on the N. side of Bishop's Itchington church, also that a stone or stones be laid over our bodies to prevent our remains being disturbed'. In 1792 the body-snatchers were certainly active, so was this a not unreasonable anxiety (despite Bishop's Itchington being some distance from any anatomy school).

Thomas Hood's doggerel poem 'Mary's Ghost', written in 1827, made light of the practice:

'Twas in the middle of the night,
To sleep young William tried,
When Mary's ghost came stealing in,
And stood at his bedside.

O William dear! O William dear!
My rest eternal ceases:
Alas! My everlasting peace
Is broken into pieces...

The body-snatchers they have come,
And made a snatch at me;
It's very hard, them kind of men
Won't let a body be!...

The arm that used to take your arm
Is took by Dr Vyse:
And both my legs are gone to walk
The hospital at Guy's...

I can't tell where my head is gone,
But Doctor Carpue can:
As for my trunk, it's all pack'd up
To go by Pickford's van.

The cock it crows – I must begone!
My William we must part!
But I'll be yours in death, altho'
Sir Astley has my heart.[13]

---

13   Thomas Hood (1799–1845), poet and humourist; Dr John Carpue, a retired army surgeon, ran a very successful private anatomical school in London; Dr Vyse is unidentified; Sir Astley Cooper we know well.

At this time, William Burke and William Hare were providing the Edinburgh anatomy school with a number of bodies, each of which attracted a payment of £7 10s., but they were eventually arrested because the bodies were suspiciously fresh: the pair were not 'resurrection men' – they had never robbed a grave in their lives – they merely murdered their victims. Hare turned King's Evidence and was pardoned, but Burke was hanged and then sent to the anatomy school for dissection – a routine procedure after capital punishment at the time. His skeleton remains on display in the School of Anatomy at Edinburgh University today.

But the future of body-snatching was to be short-lived: the trade collapsed with the passing of the Anatomy Act of 1832, which allowed unclaimed bodies from asylums, prisons and workhouses to go for dissection.

*

William Dent observed in a letter home in March 1810:

> 'The lectures in the course of six weeks will be brought to a finish and thinking myself equal to the task of being examined before the Royal College of Surgeons… this will be attended by a good deal of expense. If I pass I shall have to pay £22 for my Diploma and the other expenses attending to it.'

(Excluding an evening – at least – of celebration by the successful candidates in their favourite tavern[s], no doubt.)

Henry Lilley Smith also presented himself for examination on this date, and both candidates managed to fool the examiners. Dent wrote to his mother on 7th May 1810:

> 'I have the pleasure to inform you of my good fortune in passing my examinations on Friday night last. It has

relieved me of a great deal of anxiety I assure you and you may now congratulate yourself on having a son a MRCS which is more than most medical practitioners in the north can boast of...'[14]

'Relieved of a great deal of anxiety' indeed: the examination for Membership of the Royal College of Surgeons has always been (and remains) an extremely rigorous test of a candidate's surgical knowledge, and rightly so: 'depriving an examinee of the certificate at least prevented him from doing much harm.'[15]

A *viva* (oral) examination can go in unexpected directions: every student, in the small hours of the morning in the days before an examination, worries how he will perform.

Here is a candidate's report of his appearance for the surgical Membership:

'There were many examiners and perhaps thirty or forty students to be examined. Various questions, some very intricate, were put to the students, and success or failure in the reply at once noted. Then after a while each examiner took over one or two students for a closer examination, noting the replies as before. I was consigned to the tender mercies of a chirurgical and very eccentric knight then in great fame. He took me on a great number of subjects; and strange to say, on the treatments of most of the cases he suggested we entirely disagreed. I had been taught otherwise. I soon discovered that the worthy knight had his own crotchets upon almost everything; but in the end we got on famously. With a smile he observed, as I stuck to my teaching, "Yes, young gentleman, you answer

---

14   William Dent came from a farming family in Mickleton, in Upper Teesdale, Co. Durham.

15   Originally Dr Anthony Clare's pithy view of the hurdle of the Membership examination of the Royal College of Psychiatrists (MRCPsych).

perfectly as you have been taught in the schools, but on the field of battle and in most cases, if you adopt my plans you will do much better.'"

Fortune favours the brave.

What lay ahead for these two new Members of the Royal College of Surgeons? William Chamberlain's 'A Dissertation on the Duties of Youths Apprenticed to the Medical Profession' of 1812 forewarns fledgling surgeons of what will occasionally be among their duties to future patients:

'Are you too fine a gentleman to think of contaminating your fingers by administering a clyster [an enema] to a poor man, or a rich man, or a child dangerously ill when no nurse can be found that knows anything of the matter? This is a part of your profession that is as necessary for you to know how to perform it as it is to bleed or to dress a wound. Or are your olfactory nerves [sense of smell] too delicate that you cannot avoid turning sick when dressing an old neglected ulcer; or when, in removing dressings, your nose is assailed with the effluvia [discharge] from a carious [infected] bone? If you cannot bear these things, put surgery out of your head and go and be apprenticed to a Man Milliner or Perfumer.'

Sound advice, of course – and always a good idea to weed out the faint-hearted early on in the medical education process – but Henry and William, with some eight months of surgical practice at Colchester under their belts in addition to their instruction at Guy's and St Thomas's, were by now old hands at the game.

Once celebrations were over, and they had recovered from their hangovers, the burning question of the hour was, presumably, the one facing every newly qualified medical student: 'what now?'

Dent made up his mind quite quickly, enlisting in the army

before the end of the month. The examination for the diploma required by the Army Medical Board was less rigorous than the Membership of the College – and considerably less expensive (a mere 5s. 5d.) – so could it be William did not entirely make up his mind regarding his future career until after he had qualified MRCS, or perhaps considered the Membership would advance his army career more rapidly? Either way, come August, he was with Wellington in the Peninsula as an Assistant Surgeon to the 9th Regiment of Foot.

He plainly had a surgeon's temperament; he was to write home some years later, in June 1814:

'I am very certain that if I was settled in private practice, even superior to what I could expect, that at the expiration of a week I should wish to be in the situation I am in at present. I have a horrible dislike to be running fidgeting after a parcel of old women.'[16]

Henry Lilley Smith was more undecided: it is probable that his thoughts in Colchester of an army career were merely a passing whim – I suspect army life, especially the conversation to be had in the Officers' Mess ('… the fair sex and horses monopolised the chief part of my brother officers' thoughts and ideas', according to Dent), wasn't really for him, judging from his various pronouncements and behaviour in later years.

He appears not to have sat the Licentiate examination of the Society of Apothecaries (LSA) as well as his MRCS; many young surgeons did. The LSA, combined with the MRCS – known as 'College and Hall' – was the commonest method of entry into

---

16   Unfortunately, he was drowned at sea in 1826, whilst returning home on leave from the West Indies, where he was then stationed. After fourteen years as an Assistant Surgeon to the 9th Foot, in 1824 he had been appointed Regimental Surgeon to the 21st Foot (later the Royal Scotch Fusiliers). He was hoping to find a suitable bride in England during his forthcoming period of leave.

practice as 'surgeon, apothecary and accoucheur'[17]; the LSA allowed the holder to dispense medicines as well as prescribe them. This had been the route taken by Thomas Nicholls Adams of Walsall, and it was, at worst, a safety net should a career as a surgeon fail.

The greatest obstacle to starting in practice for any young doctor was exactly as William Dent, once again, set out in the same letter in which he had informed his mother of his success with the examiners, when returning to Mickleton was still an option for him:

> 'I know very well you are anxious to hear of my settling somewhere and I wish I could gratify you in this respect, but it does not accord with my ideas at all at present. Supposing I should come home, what is there for me to do? Even if I should begin a practice on my own account it would be several years before I could expect any established business. Another thing, my appearance is so much against me, for I am too young.'

Henry Lilley Smith applied in 1810, albeit unsuccessfully, for the post of salaried apothecary – the most junior position in the hospital – at the new Derbyshire General Infirmary. But without the LSA he was plainly not the best of candidates. So, he returned to Southam after an absence of six years – to be appointed the town's 'Parish Surgeon' in the spring of 1811.

What could Henry Lilley Smith expect on his return?

---

17   'accoucheur' = 'man-midwife', or practitioner of midwifery. They were the forerunners of today's General Practitioner.

3

RETURN TO SOUTHAM

In 1811 Southam was a small but fairly thriving market town situated at the centre of five roads that brought the traveller directly onto Market Hill. There had been a catastrophic fire in the town in February 1742, which had begun at the Craven Arms on Market Hill, destroying much of the centre of the town. A few major buildings escaped the fire: the Manor House (until recently Southam's pharmacy) and the Old Mint pub on the main street (Coventry Street) notably, and the house on the corner of Daventry Street and Wood Street, known today as the Crown Inn pub, the gable end of which clearly shows its A-frame structure and how the roofline of the once-thatched roof has been raised. Pigot & Co.'s *National Commercial Directory* of 1828 describes Southam – rather sniffily – as 'consisting of two streets, the houses forming which are arranged on the sides of the roads from Daventry to

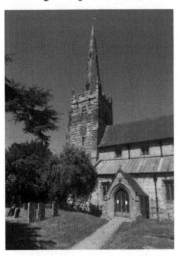

Illustration 6: All Saints Church, Ladbroke – on the south face of the tower the dial of the turret clock, made in 1818 by the Southam clockmaker Charles Oldham, is clearly visible.

Warwick and from Banbury to Coventry. The greater portion of the habitations are old and but meanly built, but the church is a neat structure having a lofty spire.'

The population in 1811 was about 1,100, mostly agricultural workers and their families, together with the usual tradesmen that every town required: blacksmith, wheelwright, thatcher, tailor, grocer (the Smith family), drapers (the Chambers family), shoemaker, clockmaker and the like.[18]

Southam had been an important stop on the drovers' road from Wales, and was also a halting place for coaches on the Chester–London and Warwick–Northampton turnpike routes and had a number of inns and hostels for travellers; the Craven Arms was the largest, providing stabling for up to eighty horses. By the 1830s eight coaches a day were stopping there.

So, now Henry had returned home to commence his medical career by 'putting up his plate' – thus advertising his presence in the town and waiting for patients to come to his door – common practice for many a young doctor; but how did he obtain the position of Parish Surgeon and what did a Parish Surgeon do?

We don't know how he managed to be appointed Parish Surgeon, but we do know how such appointments were made.

Each parish in England was responsible for the care of its poor, as required under the 1601 Poor Law, by collecting a poor-rate tax from every householder; the administration of this money was the responsibility of 'the Vestry': this was a committee, chaired by the Minister of the parish, which met monthly in the Vestry of the church and included the churchwardens and a number of unpaid 'Overseers' who were householders in the parish. Members of the Vestry were appointed annually each Easter, when the previous year's accounts were audited, following which there was usually an annual dinner.

---

18   The clockmaker was Charles Oldham, who worked in Southam from c.1770–c.1830. He made the turret clock for Ladbroke Church in 1818, for the then incumbent Revd Charles Palmer, an initial subscriber to the Infirmary and a member of the committee for many years [see Illustration 6].

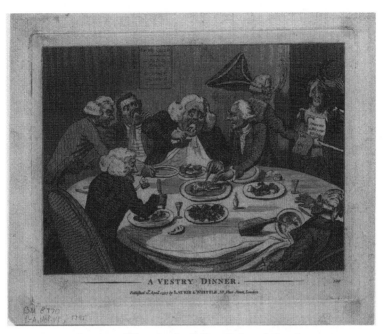

Courtesy of Chris Beetles Gallery, St James's, London
Illustration 7: 'A Vestry Dinner' – cartoon by Isaac Cruikshank, 1795.

Isaac Cruikshank sets the scene in his satirical cartoon 'A Vestry Dinner', published in 1795 [see Illustration 8]. Six noticeably well-heeled members of the Vestry are dining at a table groaning with food; an emaciated pauper stands at the threshold, holding a petition saying 'spare me a bit your worships', but is barred from entering by an attendant.

A notice on the Vestry wall behind the diners reads:

'Sit See & Say Nothing.
Eat Drink & Pay Nothing.'

An exaggeration of the Vestry's conduct, of course, but perhaps not without a grain of truth therein.

*

At this time, the Vestry would also appoint a Parish Surgeon to provide medical care for the poor of the parish, by inviting a tender from all the medical men within reach of the parish. They were, of course, seeking the lowest financial terms possible for attendance on the poor for the ensuing year, a practice known as 'farming out the poor':

> 'The parties answering are required to make an estimate of the value of their time, science, and medicines, in the relief of every disorder to which the paupers of the parish may be exposed, including the occasional inoculation or vaccination of children, and the attendance on women in labour.'

There were about 15,000 parishes in England, but some would decide to share a Parish Surgeon (who was highly unlikely to disapprove of that arrangement). Young entrants to practice locally might be able to tender quite low, but established doctors would try and block newcomers from being appointed by tendering even lower, sometimes at a financial loss, merely to obtain the post, blocking competition – and then would frequently send 'the boy' (his apprentice) to carry out the necessary treatments, whilst they themselves continued their uninterrupted attention to their private patients. The Overseers turned a blind eye to this; they were all-controlling, and would also decide – inappropriately, from a medical point of view – when to summon the doctor to attend a pauper, and could also withhold part payment of fees which they considered excessive (and did, as we shall see). Neither was there any possibility of appeal should the Vestry decide to dispense with a doctor's services (and they did, as we shall also see).

The doctors considered all this demeaning, and rightly so: a letter in the Record Office, from a Parish Surgeon to the adjoining parish's Overseers, (undated, but probably written in 1836–7) bears this out:

'Mr -----------

Overseer

Tredington

Sir,

There is a girl named Alice Cotterell, belonging to the Parish of Tredington, ill with smallpox here. I have attended her and furnished her with what was necessary – at the request of this Parish. You will do me the favour of saying whether it is your wish I should continue my attendance – the girl is still as ill as she can be.

I am,

W H Clayton

Surgeon, Blockley'

(An 'Alice Cottrill', aged fifteen, was living in Blockley in 1841, in the house of Mr & Mrs Weston and their son Charles, aged eleven, presumably as a servant. Perhaps this is the same person, now recovered from the smallpox: she would have been eleven at the time.)

Mr Clayton cannot even be bothered to ascertain the name of the Overseer in question, but merely leaves a blank scrawl, and there is no courteous salutation or valediction to his letter. Plainly the anonymous official is held in some contempt.

All this doesn't sound very confidence-inspiring to us today as regards the quality of medical care provided, and the general opinion persisted for many years that 'the attention offered to the poor by the Parish Surgeon is too often of a kind not calculated to give satisfaction'. But, in their defence, the tendering medical men were for the most part local practitioners and it would be in their best long-term interests (it would be hoped) to be seen to provide a decent standard of care as Parish Surgeons, lest their reputations – and their private practices – suffered accordingly. Let us hope so.

Medicine had limited efficacy in the Georgian era: by general opinion, surgeon–apothecaries seemed to 'do little more than use blood-letting for ailments above the midriff and purging for those below'.[19] Indeed, the author of *Therapeutics; or, the Art of Healing*, published in 1778, admitted: 'With respect to the mode of operations of medicines it must be confessed we are somewhat in the dark.'

Treatment for mental illness was worse, with certain additional physical refinements. In 1787, the year before Henry Lilley Smith was born, Edward, 5th Baron Leigh of Stoneleigh Abbey died; he had been 'pronounced lunatic' some fourteen years earlier, and had been kept at the Abbey 'under restraint' until his death.

By some fortuitous twist of fate, before being overtaken by lunacy, he had bequeathed the contents of his library at Stoneleigh to Oriel College, Oxford, where he had been an undergraduate. Oriel was then obliged to build a new library to accommodate his donation of over 1,000 titles, which were of 'unusual magnificence'.

In 1788, when King George III became mentally ill (with what is now thought to have been bipolar disorder), he was strapped to a chair, 'fixed with the eye' by the Revd Francis Willis DD, a Lincolnshire 'mad-doctor' of some repute (a Doctor of Divinity but also an Oxford MD), who then lectured him regarding self-control – the object being to scare the King into his wits, presumably.

'They beat me like a madman,' the King complained after recovery – and yet, this was the very best treatment available.

A broadside sheet published the following verse:

The King employs three doctors daily,
Willis, Heberden and Baillie,
All exceeding clever men,
Baillie, Willis and Heberden,
But doubtful which the most sure to kill is,
Baillie, Heberden or Willis.

---

19   In 1824, Byron's blood-letting by his doctors, under protest – 'more die by the lancet than by the lance' – during his last illness, which was probably malaria, resulted in a total loss of blood of about two litres (40% of the adult blood volume). No one could survive that.

The three most eminent doctors in Oxford in the early 1800s were named Wall, Pegge and Bourne; another broadsheet rhyme about those three doctors, current at the time, is amusing enough to quote:

> *I would not call in any one of them all,*
> *For only the weakest will go to the Wall;*
> *The second, like Death, that scythe-armèd mower,*
> *Will speedily make you a Pegge or two lower;*
> *While the third, with the fees he so silently earns,*
> *Is the Bourne whence the traveller never returns.*

*

By 1811, when Henry Lilley Smith returned to Southam, things weren't much better – most country surgeons practiced as apothecaries most of the time, dispensing medicines of dubious efficacy; somehow the surgeons had cornered the market in dealing with cases of venereal diseases too. One contemporary surgeon in Bristol had a discreet back entrance to his surgery, for use – after dark – by patients with such conditions.

Surgery was confined to the extremities or the more superficial areas of the body: the majority of surgical procedures carried out then could today be undertaken by any GP maintaining a surgical interest, such is the luxury of local anaesthesia: opening the chest or abdomen in the 1800s would be mortal – not that a GP today would dream of doing that either.

There is a very graphic watercolour painting with the title *'A surgical operation to remove a malignant tumour from a man's left breast and armpit in a Dublin drawing room, 1817'* which is arresting in its portrayal of surgery as it was practised in that era.

The painting is thought to have been executed by a medical student who was present at the operation. The surgeon was

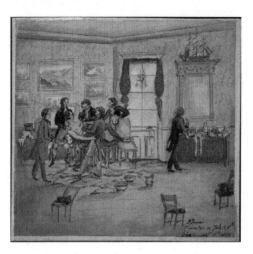

Illustration 8: 'A Surgical Operation to Remove a Malignant Tumour from a Man's Left Breast and Armpit in a Dublin Drawing Room', 1817.

Rawdon Macnamara MRCSI, then only two years qualified (he later became President of the Royal College of Surgeons in Ireland in 1831). The patient's chest wasn't opened, but the outcome was the same as if it had been for there is a handwritten note in the bottom right-hand corner informing us 'R Power Operated on July 28th Died this August 11th 1817'.

*

There are no records relating to Henry Lilley Smith's appointment, but there is a contract, of sorts, in the Record Office (such as might have existed with the Southam Parish Vestry), between the Parish Vestry at Tredington and one Edward Lyster, Surgeon, dated 5th April 1826:

'I, Edward Lyster, Surgeon, Halford Bridge, engage to attend the Parish of Tredington for one year that is to say from the 5th day of April 1826 to the 4th day of April 1827 for the sum of twenty-seven pounds – including surgery, typhus fever and general attendances – But not including Midwifery, Small Pox, Cow Pox or any outstanding paupers belonging to the Parish.'

The Tredington Parish Surgeon's contract excluded midwifery (it was probably an item-of-service payment); presumably Southam Vestry's contract was similar.

The following May, William Hornblower of Shipston-on-Stour was engaged from 24th May 1827 until 24th May 1828 'for the sum of twenty-one pounds'. Tredington Vestry could drive a very hard bargain, as we shall see.

(An itemised account for 'extras' during 'attendance upon the sick poor from April till Michaelmas at £23 per annum', submitted to the Overseers of Tredington Parish by 'H G Wells, Surgeon' in 1834 is attached [Appendix 2b]. He was summarily dismissed by the Vestry the following year – see correspondence [Appendix 3] which includes another disrespectful letter, from a different surgeon, to the Tredington Overseers).

'Outstanding paupers' probably refers to those who were in the process of claiming settlement in their present parish; this was a complicated matter whereby each parish was responsible for the persons born within it. Movement outside a parish could mean referral back to the parish of one's birth, should one fall upon hard times and need parish support soon after arrival. As Henry Lilley Smith wrote in the 2nd Annual report of the Dispensary:

'[for a labourer] to be brought home [to his own parish] for assistance would either endanger his life or deprive himself and family of that employ which kept him, and them, from the poor house, he is constrained to give up all thoughts of parochial aid, and to rely on the mercy of Heaven to send him the "good Samaritan" and the "Ladies Bountiful". '

Settlement could become the parish of one's employer, if employed by them for longer than a year – therefore servants were often employed for 364 days – or of one's spouse, if married, etc. But for a male agricultural worker to move from the parish of his birth in those days was relatively uncommon, although females entering service were more likely to. Legal costs on a parish for removal could be very high and often many times higher than the cost to the parish of maintaining the claimants in the first place – Henry Lilley Smith would argue such costs could be reduced considerably by his provident schemes, which would help keep the labouring class from calling on parish support when ill.[20]

Competition for Parish Surgeon posts was fierce; the threat often used by the Overseers to encourage low tenders from the existing practitioners was that they could easily find, for a paltry sum, 'a talented young man from the London Hospitals'.

It looks as if the Southam Vestry did just that, for there appears to have been a vacancy for Parish Surgeon at Easter 1811, following the death of the previous incumbent, according to a headstone in St James's churchyard, which bears the inscription:

'To the memory of
Bernard Geary Snow
surgeon of this place
died September 30th 1810 aged 58'

As headstones are wont to do, it also informs the reader of other unexpected events:

'Also to the memory of Frances, daughter of Bernard Geary and Rebecca Snow died 14th July 1810 aged 21 [just two months before her father]; Lucy Snow their daughter who

---

20   The annual cost in 1815 for the whole of England for litigation regarding the removal of paupers amounted to £287,000.

died 19th March 1811 aged 24 years [six months after her father]; Christiana Rolls their daughter who died March 19th 1814' [three years to the day after her sister Lucy].[21]

This information comes from records of an extensive survey of the church and churchyard made in 1916; a further survey in 1999 found many of the gravestones had since been removed from their original sites to allow for easier churchyard maintenance, or used to make boundary walls and the footpath from the 1838 lych-gate to the north door of the church. In 1999 the Bernard Geary Snow headstone was noted to have been laid flat and was partly covered by grass: it is impossible to identify it today.

Bernard Geary Snow had married Rebecca Rolls, a spinster of Bicester, in St James's Church, in 1778, after he had qualified as a surgeon from the Company of Surgeons.[22] The following year he was sufficiently established in practice as an 'apothecary and man midwife' in the town to have taken on the first of a number of apprentices, William Goode. In the absence of any records, it is my speculation that he was probably the Parish Surgeon at the time of his death, for by then he had been in practice in the town for over thirty years. He was presumably replaced by a locum until Easter 1811, when the Vestry made a new substantive annual appointment.

Another medical man suddenly appears on the scene round about this time – George Lowdell, MRCS; he is first recorded being in Southam on 27th August 1811 when he marries Jessamine Lowdell, in St James's Church, 'by special licence', since at the time of her marriage she was residing in Lingfield, Surrey; she may well have been a cousin.

---

21   I assume the three sisters all succumbed to TB: a terrible loss for the parents.

22   The Company of Surgeons had split in 1745 from the Barber-Surgeons, a City livery company established in 1540, on the insistence of the surgeons; they were granted a Royal Charter in 1800, becoming the 'Royal College of Surgeons in London', and in 1843 the 'Royal College of Surgeons of England'.

He was a Londoner and, like Henry Lilley Smith, was born in 1787. Educated at Winchester College, he appears to have managed to qualify MRCS in 1808. The only way I can explain his qualifying two years earlier than his exact contemporary is to assume (probably correctly) that Winchester's education was superior, and he entered an apprenticeship at the age of fifteen, a year earlier than Henry; and then, of course, Henry had spent most of 1809 in Colchester, which delayed his presenting himself for examination at the College of Surgeons until May 1810.

When had George Lowdell first arrived in Southam, and why? Could he have been the locum Parish Surgeon after Bernard Geary Snow's premature death? Might George Lowdell, the locum, and Henry Lilley Smith, an incomer (albeit a local boy – possibly with an influential family), have competed for the vacant position of Parish Surgeon? We just don't know. But we do know that it was the local boy – less than a year qualified and with no recorded experience in practice – whom the Vestry appointed.

We do not know if there was blood on the tracks or not, following Henry Lilley Smith's appointment as Parish Surgeon, but this did not deter George Lowdell, who continued to practice in the town in competition. Was there any animosity between the two men? Maybe, maybe not: we know that George Lowdell was a founder subscriber to the Eye Infirmary, and a committee member during his fifteen years in practice in Southam, but he didn't take up Henry Lilley Smith's offer of joining him in practice in the Dispensary. Does this reflect an uneasy truce? Possibly; Southam was a small town after all, and I suspect George Lowdell would have wanted, at the very least, to be aware of what Henry Lilley Smith was getting up to professionally.

He continued as Parish Surgeon until at least 1815 (the year of his only surviving account to the Guardian of the Poor, Southam), after which records in the Record Office are non-existent; often the position was relinquished if one's practice was well established. In any event however, after some seven years in practice in the town he must have felt he was pretty much established – with or without the continuing position of Parish Surgeon – to consider opening his own infirmary.

Many young practitioners aspired to do this; one of the first doctors to do so was William Rowley, who opened 'St John's Hospital for Diseases of the Eyes, Legs and Breasts' in Holborn, in London in 1771 – presumably those three organs were – surgically speaking – easily accessible.[23] In a pamphlet seeking voluntary contributions towards its establishment, Rowley said, '… diseases of the eyes have not been much attended to by regular practitioners, from which cause many have fell victims to the ignorant and enterprising impositions of Quacks'.

However, the hospital was not to last very long; only three years in fact. It was probably merely a mechanism for self-advertisement, given William Rowley's reputation ('his writings were calculated to promote his own private interests' said the Royal College of Physicians, despite their having awarded him membership some years earlier).

Not everyone approved of doctors opening their own hospitals; apart from the scurrilous depiction of a small provincial infirmary in the 1813 cartoon by Charles Williams, one of the more outspoken condemnations of the practice came from Thomas Wakley – who had also trained at Guy's under Astley Cooper, becoming MRCS in 1817 – when, as the editor of the medical journal *The Lancet*, which he had founded in 1828 (and

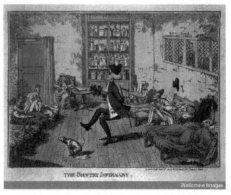

Illustration 9: 'The Country Infirmary' – cartoon by Charles Williams, 1813.

---

23   Not to be confused with 'St John's Hospital for Diseases of the Skin' in Lisle Street, Soho, founded in 1868, but absorbed into St Thomas's Hospital in 1989. The fine Lisle Street building is now a 'Slug & Lettuce' pub.

which continues to this day), he described, in 1829, personal infirmaries as 'mere nepotistic puff shops' and was scathing regarding the medical men who practised in them as being 'mostly incompetent but well-connected'; language as cutting as the name of the journal he edited. But, as with the Cruickshank and Williams cartoons, perhaps not without a grain of truth therein.

John Cunningham Saunders, born in Devon in 1773, had been apprenticed to a surgeon in Barnstaple and then attended Guy's Hospital, where he too was Astley Cooper's dresser, before becoming MRCS. After some years as Anatomy Demonstrator at Guy's, in 1804 he founded the 'London Dispensary for the Relief of the Poor Afflicted with Ear and Eye Diseases' - soon to be known as the 'London Eye Infirmary' - in rented premises (as Henry Lilley Smith would also do) in Charterhouse Square 'out of compassion for the pitiful state of many soldiers returning from the Egyptian campaign with ophthalmia'.

'Egyptian ophthalmia' concentrated orthodox doctors' minds wonderfully; it was a severe form of conjunctivitis and infection of the eye, the worst of which lasted for about two weeks, although chronic inflammation could last for months. It could also lead to scarring of the cornea and the loss of sight in one or both eyes, which would be a catastrophe for the sufferer. It first appeared during the Napoleonic wars in 1801, affected both British and French soldiers and, as conjunctivitis does in any closed community such as boarding school, it became epidemic throughout the troops rapidly. 'Spirituous liquors' and 'sexual indulgence' were blamed (both erroneously) - it was in fact a contagious disease, transmitted by touch; the sharing of towels, a common practice in the British army at the time - one towel between two soldiers - didn't help. It then spread to the civilian populations when the troops returned home.[24]

---

24   The cause is now known to be a bacterium - Chlamydia trachomatis - 'Trachoma'. Mainly a disease in children today, it is easily treated with antibiotic eye ointment and attention to general hygiene. However, it still remains the commonest cause of blindness worldwide.

Again, every cloud has a silver lining: both the Colleges of Physicians and Surgeons had heretofore disapproved of specialist practice, and the eye (and the ear) did not feature in clinical teaching at Guy's at all until about 1811. 'Egyptian ophthalmia' was to be the catalyst that made diseases of the eye respectable – and therefore a source of interest and rapidly acquired expertise by both physicians and surgeons in the nineteenth century. Hospitals for treating diseases of the eye began to appear throughout 'the Kingdom' – it helped that they were inexpensive to set up – some half dozen pre-dating Southam's Infirmary – including the Dublin Eye Infirmary (1814), which we shall look at more closely in due course.

Another of the early hospitals for diseases of the eye was the Royal Westminster Ophthalmic Hospital, founded in 1816 'for the Relief of Indigent Persons Afflicted with Diseases of the Eye' by George James Guthrie. Becoming MRCS in 1801, he then became an army surgeon in the Peninsular War; there was much eye disease among the troops in the Peninsula and so he attended a course of lectures at Cunningham Saunders' London Eye Infirmary.[25] He wrote two definitive surgical textbooks: firstly, *A Treatise on Gun-Shot Wounds and on Wounds of the Extremities Requiring the Different Operations of Amputation*, published in 1815, which ran to six editions in his lifetime (but which he considered could have been

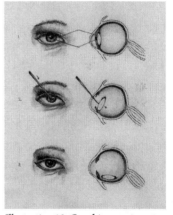

Illustration 10: Couching a cataract: the ancient operation of dislocating and displacing the lens of the eye – 'like a Smartie at the bottom of a squash ball'.

---

25   George James Guthrie (1785–1856) was apprenticed to a surgeon in Pall Mall at the age of thirteen and qualified MRCS aged sixteen: he later became Professor of Anatomy & Surgery at the Royal College of Surgeons. The Royal Westminster Eye Hospital eventually became part of Moorfields.

improved upon 'had we had another battle in the south of France, to enable me to decide two or three points of surgery which were doubtful'); and secondly, *Lectures on the Operative Surgery of the Eye* published in 1823, which ran to three editions.

Cataract surgery at that time was invariably just the ancient technique of 'couching' – from the French verb *coucher* (to lie down), displacing the lens of the eye to allow light to enter and reach the retina by merely bashing it out of position, to leave it lying like a Smartie at the bottom of a squash ball'.

However, as William Rowley stated, in England eye surgery was still usually carried out by 'irregular practitioners' – medical parlance for unqualified surgeons, who were sometimes highly skilled, sometimes not so, but 'quacks' all the same – and therefore to be avoided.

One of the more famous of the 'quack' eye surgeons was the self-styled 'Chevalier' John Taylor, who travelled throughout Europe by coach, 'couching' cataracts wherever patients were presented to him. He would usually be well away from town before the bandages were removed from patients' eyes and the occasional lamentable results of his surgery discovered – there was a high failure rate from bleeding or infection; hence the expression 'cut and run'.

The 'Chevalier' operated on the composers J S Bach in Leipzig in 1750, and G F Handel in Tunbridge Wells in 1751. Both were rendered blind; Bach died within four months of surgery, probably from infection, but Handel was luckier, living on and composing until 1759. Be all that as it may, John Taylor must have been the best of the bunch, for he was appointed oculist to King George II.

A French surgeon, Jacques Daviel, had invented a surgical technique in the 1740s for extracting the opaque lens from the interior of the eye through the cornea, which had a much more successful outcome: his technique for removing the lens of the eye (modified and refined somewhat, of course) is the basis for modern-day cataract surgery.

Inpatient facilities in the London Eye Infirmary were limited and patients were admitted only for cataract surgery; the remainder were treated as outpatients. Cunningham Saunders was a skilful surgeon and followed a refinement of Daviel's technique of extraction. He even operated on children and infants with congenital cataracts, a procedure almost unknown at the time, but apparently with some success.

A description of Cunningham Saunders' operating technique – which I will spare the reader – tells us he would 'address himself to the (restrained) patient, exhorting him to quietness, and receiving from him pretty full replies'. Quite so.

Harold Ellis FRCS, Professor of Surgery at Westminster Hospital, made this interesting observation in 1969:

'Could it be that the tradition which has died so hard in our medical schools of selecting students for their ability on the Rugby field may stem from the days when it was probably necessary to choose one's young assistants for brawn equally well as brains?'

There is a good account of surgery for cataracts in 1846 from a patient's point of view, in the days before anaesthesia, undergone by the Revd Patrick Brontë (father of Charlotte, Anne, Bramwell and Emily), at the age of seventy, in Manchester:

'Belladonna was first applied to the eye, twice, in order to expand the pupil [allowing easier access to the lens by the surgeon] – this occasioned very acute pains for only about five seconds; the feeling under the operation, which lasted fifteen minutes – was of a burning nature – but not intolerable.'

To avoid post-operative infection and bleeding into the eye, he was nursed on his back for a month with his eyes bandaged, and had leeches applied to his temples in an attempt to reduce swelling of the eye in the orbit. He wrote afterwards: 'After a year of nearly total blindness I was so far restored to sight, as to be able to read, and write, and find my way, without a guide.'

Presumably the 'not intolerable' pain was a euphemism; but an excellent recovery indeed, considering his surgery was performed with no gloves, no masks, no sterile drapes.[26] He was more fortunate than Bach or Handel.

The London Eye Infirmary flourished: in its first year it admitted 600 patients, with 500 'cured'. The next year it admitted 1,526 patients and cured 1,036; the following year, of 2,126 patients, 1,796 were cured, and so the impressive cure rate continued.

Cunningham Saunders died suddenly in 1810 from a cerebral haemorrhage, aged thirty-seven. The Eye Infirmary had been open for only five years. This was a catastrophic loss to the enterprise, but his assistants carried on his work; one, William Adams, moved to Exeter in 1808 where he opened the first eye infirmary in the provinces – Henry Lilley Smith's opened in 1818.

The London Infirmary moved to a new building in Upper Moorfields in 1824, and was renamed the London Ophthalmological Infirmary: today it is known as Moorfields Eye Hospital, and has an international reputation for excellence.

Like William Rowley and Cunningham Saunders, Henry also decided to limit his sphere of hospital practice.

---

26   In 1856, cocaine in solution eye drops, which anaesthetised the cornea, were introduced into surgical practice: this allowed the patient to co-operate by lying still with an open eye, much reducing the necessity of physical restraint.

4

THE INFIRMARY FOR THE TREATMENT OF DISEASES OF THE EYE AND EAR

On 13th April, 1818, at a meeting in the Craven Arms Inn in Southam, Henry Lilley Smith presented his 'Prospectus for the Establishment of the Nature of an Infirmary on a small scale and at a moderate expense in Southam in the County of Warwick, for the benefit of the Poor, afflicted with diseases of the Eye and Ear'.

Although Cunningham Saunders died in 1810, Henry Lilley Smith claimed to have known him whilst in London, stating in his prospectus that he had practised in Southam 'the improved methods of his friend Mr Saunders for seven years'.

He set out his requirements in the prospectus, as its 'Oculist and Aurist', which, considering that the building he proposed to use was already available, gives a good indication of the working Infirmary once established: 'Three rooms in a small house, a vapour bath, a galvanic trough, electric apparatus, some few instruments etc.,' and he comments that '... diseases of the Eye and Ear are a highly interesting class of diseases, and the disorders with which the poor are afflicted usually arise from accidental causes connected with their employment, over which they have no control, and as they rarely engage the attention of medical men visiting the parochial class [paupers], the patient is induced to use a few domestic remedies, which generally do harm, and the cases become chronic.'

He continued: 'Many eye accidents befall labourers cutting hedges, breaking stones on the road, hoeing turnips etc and are prevented from becoming burdens on the Parish by their treatment and cure.' Moreover, he notes, 'Patients afflicted with these diseases are not prevented from travelling, and they will readily attend where they have a prospect of relief.' (And travel they did.)

Most small infirmaries and hospitals were financed by a combination of charitable donations and subscriptions.[27] Annual subscribers of one guinea and benefactors of five guineas and upwards to the Southam Infirmary had the right to admit two patients annually; annual subscribers of half a guinea, one patient. Each admission could remain 'at the expense of the funds' for a maximum of two months.

A patient seeking admission – as was very much the case with all charitable medical institutions at the time – would therefore have to beg, borrow or steal a ticket from an individual subscriber, and make his case for being a 'proper object of charitable care', which didn't necessarily depend on the urgency of any individual case.

Running costs were kept modest by Henry Lilley Smith providing medical care *gratis*, and the Infirmary providing merely 'a bed and all necessary medication'; patients had to pay for their board, initially for 9d. per week (8d. if female and 6d. if aged under ten years) and patients admitted had to provide themselves with '2 shirts, 2 pairs stockings & 2 night-caps'. Paying for one's own board and lodging was a shrewd move: it encouraged early discharge from the hospital.

---

27   It was Sir Astley Cooper, in fact, who opened the first cottage hospital – the West Herts Infirmary – in Piccotts End, Hertfordshire, in 1827.

The chairman of the meeting in the Craven Arms was Sir Gray Skipwith, Baronet and J.P., who had been instrumental in establishing Southam's charity school.[28] He also took much interest in the provision of medical treatment in Warwickshire, and helped to raise funds by attending annual charity balls held in aid of the dispensaries established (on traditional charitable lines) in Stratford-upon-Avon in 1823 and in Warwick in 1826 by Dr John Conolly, then a Stratford-upon-Avon general practitioner.

The medical men appointed were Henry Lilley Smith, as surgeon, together with four honorary physicians, Charles Rattray MD of Daventry, Charles Wake MD of Warwick, Peter Francis Luard MD of Warwick, and Amos Middleton MD of Leamington, who could be consulted should the need arise with tricky cases, and who would also have given their services *gratis*. (When Dr Amos Middleton opened a small infirmary and dispensary in Leamington in 1824, Henry Lilley Smith was likewise appointed its honorary 'Oculist'.)

Sir Gray Skipwith was appointed President, and the Infirmary was to be run by a committee of twenty, appointed from the Patrons, President, Vice-Presidents (twenty), and Treasurer. Of the initial 157 donors and subscribers, there were four members of the aristocracy (lords, earls etc.), four knights of the realm, six physicians, nine surgeons, twenty-six clergy and forty-six esquires (these included all the surgeons but none of the physicians – a subtle stratification of class here, I suspect), and W L Smith and Henry Chambers (Henry Lilley Smith's father and maternal grandfather); the surgeons were mostly from the surrounding district, but also from as far distant as Rugby, Long Buckby, Banbury and Hinckley – all very much as one would expect for such a project.

One benefactor of five gns and an initial subscriber was 'F. Dwarris, Esq. London'. This was Fortunatus Dwarris; Henry's father had an elder sister, Sarah, who married a Warwick man

---

28   Recorder of Stratford-upon-Avon 1823–1835 & MP 1831–1835. He was descended through his mother's side from the American Indian princess Pocohontas; d. Hampton Lucy, 1852, survived by at least fifteen of his twenty children.

with lands in the West Indies, William Dwarris, and they had a son some five years later, christened Fortunatus William Lilley Dwarris, who by this time was a lawyer in London.[29] He and Henry Lilley Smith were cousins, hence his support.

The building utilised was owned by his father, as was the adjoining house and gardens in which Henry Lilley Smith later lived with his family.[30] From deeds in the Record Office it can be ascertained that the building which was to become the Infirmary had been acquired by Henry's father, William Lilley Smith, in 1808, from its owners William Basse (the Parish Clerk) and George Pearson (Henry's mother's uncle; he of the body-snatching anxieties) – but when it had been originally built and for what purpose is not known. However, by June, the Infirmary was up and running, with fourteen beds, a resident matron and a domestic servant. Nursing experience or practice was not then

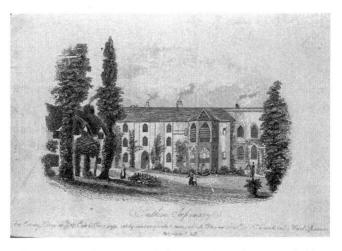

Illustration 11: The Eye & Ear Infirmary c.1850 – drawing probably by Sophia Smith

29   Fortunatus William Lilley Dwarris (1786–1860); educated at Rugby School and Oxford, and entered the Middle Temple in 1811. He was knighted in 1838 for services to a Royal Commission.

30   All of which were bequeathed to him on his father's death in 1844.

part of a Matron's duties; they were entirely administrative and in her domain she ruled supreme – an American visitor to a hospital in England a hundred years later commented, 'the title of Matron suggests in England dignity only a little less than that of the Prime Minister's' – her powers today are, regrettably, much diminished.

A notice published, 'By Order of the Committee', on 7th June, set out the Infirmary's aims and objectives:

> 'This Institution offers advice, medicine, lodgings, and nursing, gratuitously, when recommended by a subscriber, and as constitutional disease forms a very considerable part of those complaints which impair the sight and hearing, the vicinity of Southam to the saline springs of Leamington, will, on that account, be found peculiarly advantageous...'

Leamington Priors, then merely a village some two miles from Warwick, the county town, was to find that its 'saline springs' would revolutionise its fortunes. The Pump Rooms, built in 1814, provided treatment in 'twenty baths of every description' for the many patients who visited the town as its reputation as a spa grew. The very elegant 'Turkish hammam' room is still visitable, being now part of Leamington Museum.

The waters, which taste ghastly, also have a mild laxative effect (of course), so 'taking the waters' internally was encouraged by the town's physicians.[31] Indeed, those who took the waters 'injudiciously', i.e. without first seeking professional medical advice as to dose and frequency – 'water bibbers' – were very much discouraged.[32] Spa towns were recommended for so many diverse medical conditions, including 'phthisis' (TB of the lungs), that it

---

31   See Appendix 6 for a description of a typical prescription by Dr Amos Middleton for a patient.

32   A tap dispensing water *gratis* from Leamington's still functioning spring can be found today adjacent to the Royal Pump Rooms. It still tastes ghastly.

seems to me the doctors, by recommending 'taking the waters' so enthusiastically as they did, were, in essence, behaving little differently from the 'quacks' whom they so despised; but no matter.

In 1826 *A Visitor's Guide to Leamington* made the comment: 'Leamington, instead of continuing a struggling village inhabited by peasantry in the winter, and in the summer only by a few invalids is now become the resort of elegance and fashion.'[33]

Surprisingly, despite the reference to Leamington's newly promoted reputation as a spa, there is no mention by Henry Lilley Smith of Southam's ancient Holy Well, a spring just to the east of the town, with alleged healing powers, particularly for eye ailments – perhaps because the spring water is intensely cold. It is extremely unlikely that this local source of pure, cold, water close to the Infirmary would have been overlooked; almost certainly it would have been utilised on a daily basis. Unlikely not to have been. It is now a Scheduled Ancient Monument and

Grade ll listed building, and it had been excluded from the 1761 Enclosure Act, with the proviso that it be fenced with oak posts and rails, with free access for all Southam inhabitants. And so it remains today; to visit it is a pleasant walk beside the River Stowe – but today the

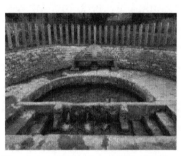

Illustration 12: Southam's Holy Well (once the only source of water for the town)

housing estate monster is creeping ever closer.

Financially, the annual subscribers produced enough income to cover expenditure for bed and medication each year, which was surprisingly unchanged throughout most of the years of

---

33   The population of Leamington Priors in 1811 was 543; by 1830 it was 6,000, and ten years later was double that. It was the making of Dr Henry Jephson MD, a local physician (or perhaps he was the making of Leamington); his fashionable medical practice, which involved much bathing in and 'taking of' the waters, brought him and the town a fortune.

its operation during Henry Lilley Smith's lifetime (about £120/ annum – he had initially projected costs would be about £80/ annum). Benefactors presumably offset starting costs involved with the building, and further donations would have always been welcome to help defray the household costs. Such institutions found these occasionally came from unexpected sources; one donation recorded for the London Eye Infirmary was '1 guinea – found on the table', and a donation of £5 for the Southam Infirmary had originally been 'Paid by the Proprietors of the Bristol Coach to the Reverend W. Morgan, of Stockton, and Charles Harwood Esq. of Southam, for being negligently and furiously driven', which they graciously forwarded on to the Infirmary.

The Royal Dispensary for Treatment of Diseases of the Ear in Dean Street, Soho (established in 1815) frequently received substantial amounts from collections made after sermons preached in fashionable London churches, but Henry Lilley Smith disapproved of the practice, certainly with regard to his Infirmary, adding the following comment to the Infirmary's annual report of 1857 – which would prove to be his last: 'It should be observed, that from the beginning no Sermon has been preached and no Ball nor Bazaar held in its behalf.'

The Infirmary continued to flourish; an abstract of the 12th Annual Report of the Infirmary of 1st July 1830 was published in the *Northampton Mercury* newspaper and other 'country newspapers', and is worth closer study, as it gives an idea of how the Infirmary was performing just over ten years after it had opened.

Sir Gray Skipwith continued to be President, but the number of honorary physicians had increased to eight – the original four plus George Mellor MD and Joseph Rann MD, both of Coventry, Archibald Robertson MD of Northampton and John Conolly MD, now of London.[34]

---

34   Conolly had left Stratford-upon-Avon in 1828 to become the first Professor of Medicine at University College London. He resigned after two years and returned to a house in Theatre Street, Warwick, until his final move to Hanwell Asylum in 1839.

Whereas the Infirmary's original committee of twenty had included four members of the clergy, the committee now included fifteen: this is surprising, for the obituary of Henry Lilley Smith in the *Leamington Spa Courier* comments that 'many of the clergy of the district stood aloof from the Infirmary and denounced his principles'. Perhaps he was to alienate them in his later years.

In the previous twelve months, 283 patients had been admitted (253 with eye conditions; thirty with ear conditions) of whom 168 were cured and seventy relieved. The total number of patients treated since the Infirmary opened was 3,138.

It was financially secure, with a surplus for the previous year of £123 14s 10d. Payment for board had increased to 6 shillings per week (5 shillings if female and 4 shillings or 3/6d. if a child).

The abstract of the 1830 Annual Report contained a complete list of subscribers – this was deliberate:

'Overseers of Parishes and benevolent Individuals desirous of sending patients, may be acquainted with the Names of Subscribers who have a right to grant them admission tickets; hitherto, for want of the Public having this information, some Subscribers have not used their tickets at all, whilst others have become the medium by which as many as Thirty Patients have been sent in one year to the Infirmary.'

A comparison of the list of subscribers from 1818 with the list of 1830 shows some interesting differences. An overview will suffice; only six physicians were subscribers in 1818, but by 1830 there were ten, and now included Dr Henry Jephson MD.

In 1818 only two parishes became subscribers: Southam parish (sensibly), and the 'directors of the poor for Coventry'. In 1830 seven parishes had admitting rights: Braunston, St Michael's Coventry, Holy Trinity Coventry, Chilvers Coton, Draycott, Foleshill and Meriden. But not Southam – odd.

The occupants of a number of nearby 'big houses' subscribed in 1818: Packington Hall, Ragley Hall, Farnborough Hall, Walton Hall, Upton Hall, Shuckborough Hall, Guy's Cliffe and Warwick Castle. By 1830, there were twelve, and the net had extended wider afield to include newcomers Charlecote, Stoneleigh Abbey, Fawsley Hall and Althorp.

There was some pressure on the Infirmary to provide treatment as the years passed: so much so that in 1840 it was decided by the committee to permit the clergy to recommend poor persons for outpatient treatment, without limit and without payment; clergy were also circulated to a radius of fifteen miles of Warwick and Northampton with a list of subscribers who could make application for inpatient treatment on behalf of deserving parishioners.

Patients from far afield would often present themselves at the Infirmary (presumably having obtained a ticket of admission from one of the distant subscribers), only to find that for one reason or another they were unsuitable; either their eye conditions were beyond any possible treatment or because of the requirement that all admissions to the Infirmary be 'proper objects of charity; no persons to be deemed objects but such as are necessitous'. Henry Lilley Smith became irritated by – to use his own expression – 'the wearers of gaudy clothes' (those well able to afford doctors' fees) obtaining recommendations for admission from subscribers. To prevent this Henry Lilley Smith began to hold 'outpatient clinics' in surrounding towns on their market days, and see patients referred to him to decide, for one reason or another, if they were suitable cases for treatment, and follow up as necessary those who had been discharged. For example, the *Northampton Mercury* for 24th August 1822 had the following announcement among the 'small ads':

'Mr Smith, Member of the Royal College of Surgeons of London – Oculist and Aurist to the Infirmary at Southam, Warwickshire, for curing Diseases of the EYE and EAR, will attend at the George Inn, Northampton, on the First and Third Tuesday of every month.

Subscribers to the Infirmary in the Vicinity of Northampton sending Patients, with recommendations, to see Mr Smith at the George Inn, are requested to desire them to attend exactly at Twelve o'clock.'

He also held clinics weekly on a Saturday at the Warwick Arms, Warwick, and monthly at the Eagle Hotel, Rugby, and at 'Mrs Claridge's, High Street, Banbury'. How did he travel to them?

It has been said that the definitive social history of the rural general practitioner and his horse has yet to be written (regrettably, this is not it).

The Horse-World of London in 1893 considered that 'the doctor's horse was his most important asset; it had to be chosen for stamina and sound temperament, look none the worse for standing about in the rain, and it helped if it also had the intelligence to be capable of trundling home late at night, with its exhausted master fast asleep in the saddle': a mettlesome hunter, however elegant, would soon disappoint.

'My riding today upon account of visiting has been upwards of 20 miles or near 30. Lord bless me and the beast I ride upon,' a rural practitioner wrote in his diary.

'Horse-World' again: '… many a one-horse doctor walks his round on Sunday to give his weary steed a rest'.[35]

Sir Walter Scott said of the (fictional) rural surgeon-apothecary Dr Gideon Gray in his 1827 novel *The Surgeon's Daughter*: 'There is no creature in Scotland that works harder and is more poorly requited than the country doctor, unless, perhaps, it be his horse.' Dr Gray was said to cover 5,000 miles a year on

---

35   Dr Frank Smorfitt, a general practitioner in Southam from 1931 until his death in 1977, rider-to-hounds and amateur horse breeder (notably of 'Santa Claus', winner of the 1964 Derby), was still making house visits to patients in the 1950s on horseback – occasionally wearing hunting pink, according to some patients.

horseback: for this he required two horses – Mortar and Pestle – 'which he exercised alternately' – a kindness, if an expensive one.

Henry Lilley Smith almost certainly also made his visits to patients in Southam and the surrounding villages on horseback (we know his house had a stable and gardens) – but for such return journeys as these – Warwick, twenty-two miles; Rugby, twenty-two miles; Banbury, twenty-eight miles; Northampton, forty-six miles – and 'commencing consultations at twelve o'clock exactly' – he would probably have travelled by dog-cart (actually horse-drawn: it was so-called because sporting dogs could be kept in a box behind the driver) or some other form of single carriage, or possibly by one of the mail coaches ('with interior seating for four travellers') that travelled to all the above towns via the improved turnpike roads of the early 1800s, although I can't see Henry Lilley Smith in a mail coach, somehow. (Dr Henry Parsey, of Hatton Asylum, had in the 1860s his own very fine four-wheeled carriage, together with a coachman, a rehabilitated ex-patient.)

The *Northampton Mercury* advertisement appeared for over thirty years; apparently these clinics did not endear him to the local medical practitioners, who felt that he was also taking the opportunity to 'poach' fee-paying patients from their practices, in addition to treating the 'labouring poor' referred by local subscribers to the Infirmary. Whether this was true or not, Henry Lilley Smith robustly denied it, claiming he was 'supplying a deficiency which they had not even perceived, and that the moment they could do the work he was doing, he would retire'. He didn't.

But then, general practitioners have always been sensitive to the practice of 'poaching' by rivals, and probably especially so then, with the rapidly increasing numbers of military and naval doctors looking to set up in civilian practice after the end of the Napoleonic wars. It would have been highly unlikely not to have happened at all. A consultation fee is a consultation fee is a consultation fee. And besides, Henry Lilley Smith was well conversant with the families in the local 'big houses', and his obituary in the *Leamington Spa Courier* (Leamington's first newspaper, founded in 1828) reported that he was 'suave in deportment' – he could, no doubt, cut a dash with 'the higher classes' should the prospect of a private consultation (and fee) present itself.

Over the years, admission of diseases of the ear to the Infirmary became increasingly infrequent. Henry Lilley Smith said in his report of 1857:

'Disorders of the ear are less numerous than disorders of the eye, and less easy to be cured... but even where complete cures were not obtained or expected, symptoms have been removed which are known to frequently precede serious and fatal disorders: and young persons labouring under deafness from peculiar causes have so far been cured as to be capable of receiving instruction at school, and of taking and keeping services, to which they would otherwise have been quite unequal.'

The interior of the ear could only be examined with difficulty, using a polished silver speculum and reflected daylight for illumination (ideally), or candlelight aided by various optical lens contraptions (less so); this meant diagnosis and surgical treatment was limited, and treatment was still, for the most part, rudimentary. Those with discharging ears (and there would have been a good number, often children) in the pre-antibiotic era, would have had to re-attend frequently to have their ear canals carefully painted with a dilute silver nitrate solution – an early antiseptic. For some this attention would have been prolonged and tedious, for patient and doctor both – perhaps with an occasional leeching for good measure – and before treatment was completed often 'both patient and practitioner would be well tired of each other'.[36]

---

36   The view of Sir William Wilde FRCSI (1815–1876): a distinguished Irish eye and ear surgeon and father of the more famous Oscar.

Although the ear conditions that required admission to the Infirmary were not classified as carefully as the eye conditions, it is probable that Henry Lilley Smith treated many conditions of the ear in his surgery, and not in the Infirmary.

We know that, like any other country doctor, he treated urgencies and emergencies as the necessity arose: his solitary surviving account to Southam's Guardian of the Poor for the first quarter of 1815 for his Parish Surgeon duties had included attending a miscarriage and lancing abscesses of the foot and breast (in two different patients); and when on 14th December 1829 an itinerant tinker woman travelling on the Warwick Road out of Southam was robbed and assaulted close to the Infirmary, she was taken to his surgery where she received 'every assistance that skill and humanity could suggest', according to the report in the *Leamington Spa Courier* of 26th December. He would surely have found it impossible not to attend to them as circumstances demanded; his reputation (and income) would have suffered – and, after all, he professed himself to be an 'Oculist and Aurist'.

One of few surgeons of the period (along with Cunningham Saunders) to take any interest in diseases of the ear was Astley Cooper, and this may well have influenced Henry Lilley Smith whilst he was his dresser at Guy's; in 1801 Astley Cooper had restored the hearing in two patients by perforating the eardrum (myringotomy), but he was highly selective in his choice of patients – the cause of deafness had to be demonstrated to be due to fluid within the middle ear and not nerve damage (which was, of course, irremediable). Other surgeons then attempted likewise to restore hearing by myringotomy, but were less successful; they were probably not as selective, or they sometimes caused inadvertent damage to the anatomy of the inner ear beyond the eardrum, or introduced infection – which made things worse rather than better. The procedure then fell out of favour until taken up again after Henry Lilley Smith's lifetime, notably by Sir William Wilde, but only because by then advances in the diagnosis of the presence of fluid behind the eardrum allowed him to be meticulous in his selection of suitable patients.

The County Record Office holds a letter from a certain Lady Amherst, about her severe earache of many months, written on 31st May 1813; she suffered leeches and 'cupping' – the same treatment as meted out to Byron in 1824 (but not for earache) – calomel purges (of course), and 'electricity', but none was effective. She wrote:

> 'A surgeon of great eminence advised a plaister comprised of half an ounce of Cienta [knotgrass, apparently] and a quarter of an ounce of opium/hemlock and opium… well mixed together and spread upon some Apothecary's sticking plaister of a size nearly of a crown piece and left on till it drops off.
>
> A quarter of an hour after I applied it I found relief and in an hour I was well, but strange to tell that night when it fell off in my sleep the pain returned, on putting on the plaister it again subsided.'[37]

Therapeutics hasn't changed much – patches applied to the skin are a convenient method of drug delivery still in use.

Diseases of the eye which Henry Lilley Smith treated appear to have been mainly inflammatory and infective conjunctivitis (there was still some 'Egyptian ophthalmia' around), and corneal ulceration; some surgery was performed, but this was restricted to repairing injury and conditions pertaining to the eyelids (inverted and everted eyelashes, and tumours of the eyelid, etc.); operation on the eye for cataract seems to have been very infrequent.

According to Cunningham Saunders' *Manual of Treatment of Diseases of the Eye*, infective conditions of the eye would need prolonged bathing and frequent applications of various

---

37   Little more is known about her; she may have introduced into the UK from China the elegant 'Lady Amherst's pheasant' (*Chrysolophus amherstiae*) as a game bird in 1828, which is now almost extinct.

eye drops (dilute silver nitrate again) for perhaps two to three weeks. Internal inflammatory disorders of the eyeball ('iritis' etc.) were – and still are – much more serious conditions, and would require leeches or blood-letting from the temporal artery (not much fun) in addition. Treatment invariably included ensuring the 'free elimination of the toxins which have accumulated in the blood'; Cunningham Saunders advised 'jalap 2 scruples daily' (one doesn't need much imagination to know what effect that produced).

How did the work Henry Lilley Smith carried out compare with elsewhere? The best comparison that I could find is with Dublin's Eye Infirmary (est. 1814): the diagnostic classifications are almost identical. Despite Southam's only available published list being from 1831–2 and Dublin's from 1814–17, and the overall numbers treated in Dublin being very much greater (2,840) compared to Southam (311), the conditions treated are very similar in proportion, with infectious disorders being the majority of cases and cataract surgery being very limited indeed in both hospitals. Dublin treated no patients with diseases of the ear, and Southam doesn't list children separately – although children were included in the tariff of charges for board, so were probably included in the overall numbers. The comparison – which can appear a bit technical – can be seen in Appendix 5.

Henry Lilley Smith was quite transparent about the work the Infirmary carried out. He repeatedly invited interested parties to Southam, 'to witness the management of the Southam Dispensary for a period of three months: and it is probable that young medical practitioners, or those about to commence practice [who would also have an opportunity of visiting the Eye and Ear Infirmary], will find it advantageous to avail themselves of this offer.'

*

With the Infirmary established, Henry Lilley Smith must have considered he was financially secure; secure enough in any event to marry a Southam girl, Mary Bicknell, in St James's Church on 2nd October 1819; his son William would later write 'both my parents' families for at least three or four generations had been born at, or intimately connected with, the town.'

Born on 29th October 1793, she was the daughter of Thomas Bicknell, a gentleman farmer and his wife Sarah; she was six years Henry's junior.

They went on to have three children together: their first child, Henry Chambers Smith (baptised in St James's on 4th August 1824), died aged nine months on 14th May 1825 and was buried in the family tomb; the second, William Lilley Smith (born 7th August 1826), was sent to Westminster School in London (where he rowed in the school eight versus Eton), and then to Trinity College, Cambridge, in 1845 graduating BA in 1849. He was then ordained in 1850 and spent his life in the Church, becoming Rector of Dorsington, near Stratford-upon-Avon, in 1866. He never married.

Their youngest child, Mary Sophia Smith (known as 'Sophia'), was baptised in St James's on 7th January 1836. She seems to have been a somewhat shadowy, reclusive member of the family; the only information which could be found regarding her activities in life is that she was an accomplished artist: she made the pen and ink drawings of Southam which illustrated her brother's book (see later), and made another collection of similar drawings of various manor houses and churches in the Stratford-upon-Avon area in 1870–71, which were found in 1911 in a manuscript book which had belonged to Robert Fisher Tomes (1823–1904), a farmer and amateur zoologist of Long Marston; it is presumed he was going to add commentaries in the intervening pages, but this never happened.

They are very attractive drawings: some have provided illustrations to this book.

She appears to have lived in Southam for most of her life, although in 1851, aged fifteen, she was living for an unknown period as a 'collegian' (and doing what, exactly?) in the house in Portland Place of William MacIntyre MD, physician to the Western General Dispensary in Lisson Grove, London.[38] She does not appear to have pursued a career as such as an artist – traceable works of hers are limited to only those described in this book.

At some date after 1851, she returned to Southam to live with her mother, and they lived their last years with her brother William, in the Rectory at Dorsington.

From the details of her death certificate, her occupation was given as 'proprietor of land and houses', so presumably the family's property brought her in a private income.

---

38   William MacIntyre MD (Edin), FRCP (1792–1857), a native of Inverness, was for many years consulting physician to the Western General Dispensary in Lisson Grove, NW8, established in 1830 as a charitable institution – the local populace being considered too poor to afford the contributions required for a provident dispensary. In 1936, it amalgamated with the St Marylebone General Dispensary.

5

THE PROVIDENT DISPENSARY

The year following the opening of the Infirmary Henry Lilley Smith published a pamphlet on 1st March 1819 entitled *Observation on the Prevailing Practice of Supplying Medical Assistance to the Poor, commonly called the Farming of Parishes; with Suggestions for the Establishment of Parochial Medicine Chests; or Infirmaries in Agricultural Districts*, addressed to 'The Patrons, President, Vice-Presidents, and Governors of the Eye and Ear Infirmary, established in the Town of Southam April 13, 1818'. In this, after a preamble regarding the failings, as he saw them, of the Vestry's practice of 'farming out' medical care to the poor, he proposed a plan for establishing a Dispensary open to all the 'labouring poor', and also the paupers of the parish – if recommended by the Overseers.

The cost of illness was an ever-present anxiety to the labourer. In 1787, one commentator wrote:

'The apothecaries in the country charge so highly for their attendance and medicines that a poor distressed hardworking man (if he is a few weeks into illness) dreads the consequences of employing him as if he survives the illness he knows it will be an additional drawback in his labour (for perhaps several years) to get clear of the apothecary.'

The relationship between doctors and clergy appears to have been one of wariness; it is noteworthy that of the ninety-six donors to Henry Lilley Smith's Memorial Fund (of which more later) thirty-one were from the clergy, but their donations amounted to a mere 3% of the total sum collected. The ever-forthright Thomas Wakley published a letter in *The Lancet* from a disillusioned Parish Surgeon in Sheffield who claimed:

'Medical men debase themselves to become the mere tools of a few clergymen, who preach up charity and good works, but never themselves work for nothing. The medical man, at whose expense others are so very charitable... is treated like a dog... In every sense these jobs are a curse to society and not blessings.'

Thus the concept of 'provident dispensaries' was launched. His dispensary would provide outpatient medical care for two classes of patients: agricultural workers and the servant class within a radius of six miles of Southam (making home visiting a viable proposition), who would claim treatment via their own subscriptions, together with paupers dependent on the parish, for whom the Vestry would make a *pro rata* contribution (at an agreed rate). Palliative care for the dying from cancer and TB would be included in the care provided. (Parish Surgeons were ordinarily not required to attend such cases.)

Funding would come from three sources: charitable donations, individual subscriptions and the Vestry. This policy differed from the Infirmary, where annual subscribers received admission tickets to give to those patients they sponsored for treatment.

Each subscription would be 3s 6d for an adult and 2s for a child under fifteen per year.[39]

Midwifery, an integral part of the practice of a country doctor, was surprisingly not included, but provision would have had to be made somehow, in any event. Presumably it was an additional item of service, attracting a fee if a Dispensary doctor was summoned to a delivery (as was the case with most other dispensaries established later).

The premises were already in existence and adjacent to the Infirmary – the thatched two-storey cottage is clearly visible behind the two poplar trees on the left in the illustration taken from a prospectus of the Dispensary (and subject to a little poetic licence in the name of marketing I suspect, if compared to the other drawing by Sophia Smith in Illustration 11). It had previously been the residence of William Basse, the Parish Clerk who had witnessed William Lilley Smith's marriage and who had later sold him the Infirmary premises.

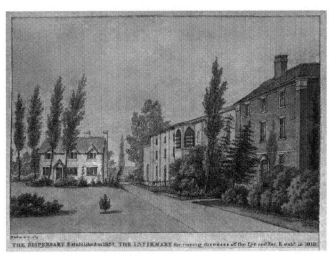

Illustration 13: The Dispensary and The Infirmary c.1823

39　　　At that rate, two parents and two children would be covered for medical care *per annum* for the equivalent of 1p/week today.

The author of a handwritten article (undated) in the Southam Heritage Collection comments that 'a certain Mrs R Wilmott, who lived at "Walton's Close", a bungalow in Watton's Lane, stated Watton's Lane should be called Walton's Lane, after the first dispenser who lived in the Dispensary Cottage, which once stood in front of where her bungalow now stands [and where Cedarlea Dental Surgery is now sited].'

The first provident dispensary 'in the Kingdom' opened in 1823. Henry Lilley Smith was indefatigable (and ever the optimist) in promoting what he – rightly – considered to be a *modus operandi* of providing better medical care to the poor in a more dignified – and less expensive – manner than that provided by the Parish. He even tried to gain the support of the House of Commons for the provision of provident dispensaries by sending a petition there on 14th April 1824. He wound up his petition thus:

'In conclusion, your petitioner further declares, that it is constant with his belief, as well as in some degree with his actual knowledge, that if the sums paid by parishes according to their contracts; with such sums as they pay on account of unforeseen cases, not included in them; together with the various sums collected from the poor for that medical assistance which to themselves appears the most cheap and efficacious, were judiciously employed in the formation of District Dispensaries [run on his provident dispensary principles], they might be provided without distressing their best feelings in regard to independence, at their own homes, or at the Dispensary; which would assure the most speedy and effectual re-establishment of health, combining likewise, when it might be necessary, the skill of all the practitioners within the district, and promoting unanimity amongst the profession, whilst in all probability it would ultimately remove one third of the pauper population from the parochial funds.

Therefore your petitioner prays this Honourable House, that the subject in all its various bearings, be forthwith be referred to the consideration of a committee of the House.

H. L. Smith'

However, provident dispensaries would only come to be adopted as 'best practice' long after his lifetime.

Lilley Smith was a radical thinker in other ways too, advocating that general practitioners pooled their skills and abilities: this idea, again, would have to await the introduction of the NHS before 'group practice' within a single building became policy, and entrenched competition between (single-handed) practitioners was – partly, at least – abolished.

The philosophy behind the provident dispensary *per se* was not, of course, new. Because hospitals were selective in the illnesses they would admit – invariably sufferers from epilepsy, insanity, cancer, TB and infectious (including venereal) diseases were declined admission – and they were often some distance away in any event other more local support services were required in rural areas. Many small 'Penny Clubs', administered at parochial level and often involving local clergy, were formed to partly remedy this lack: weekly allowances would be collected from members with the object of providing either some income in sickness and a sum of money to bury a deceased member or his wife (or child), or for shoes for the children, or to provide linen and baby clothing for women in the weeks following childbirth. (There are no records surviving of the 'Warwick Lying-In Society', but Appendix 8 has the administrative details of the 'Hungerford Lying-In Charity', which would probably have been similar in most respects.)

One of the earliest of such local benefit clubs – by the end of the 1800s there would be some 30,000 nationally – was 'The Fountain of Hospitality', a Friendly Society begun by Benjamin Satchwell, of Leamington, in 1777. Its members were 'united in a band of peace and goodwill, to glorify God, to comfort and assist each other as Christian Brethren, to provide for the sick, the lame, the blind, the prisoners, the widows, the orphans, the infirmities of old age, and to bury the dead.[40] Quite a task.

The organisers of most benefit clubs would hold monthly meetings, often in a room in a local pub, and, at the annual 'reckoning', if there was a surplus then it was usual practice to establish a reserve fund (of about 1s per member), with any additional funds remaining distributed to the members. This might well be an occasion for some overindulgence – a pattern of behaviour of which Henry Lilley Smith disapproved, as we shall discover. His proposal of 'Alfred Societies' was much more decorous.

Although his repeated invitation to 'all and every regular Medical Practitioner in the District to become admitted to the Establishment' and take part in providing medical care from the Dispensary, if they so wished, none did so. Why that was is not known; his concept of the self-supporting dispensary was not well accepted by some local colleagues; perhaps there was a continued underlying resentment of the manner of his arrival in Southam – he once said he had 'come to Southam almost as a stranger'; not entirely true, of course – or that a dispensary would upset the *status quo* of the other medical men in the town, reducing their practices and thus their income. Then again, it may have been because of his demeanour and the brusque language he tended to use, which his obituary (diplomatically) described as 'trifling defects of language'. This extract from the Second Annual Report of the Southam Dispensary will suffice as an example:

'Centripedal Dispensaries [as he sometimes referred to provident dispensaries in their early years], on the other hand, will have the advantage of giving immediate

---

40   Benjamin Satchwell (1732–1810) also contributed to the development of Leamington as a spa, by forming a charity in 1806 which provided accommodation and saline baths for the sick poor at 'Abbott's Spa' in Bath Street, long since demolished.

medical relief, and of thus frequently arresting progress or diminishing the violence of a serious complaint. They will render less frequent the necessity of parochial aid, and in this way at once prevent an increase of expense to the parish – and do away with the necessity of *dealing wholesale with the bowels of the sick poor* [his italics] – as well as keep up in the mind of the poor man that honest, useful, and laudable spirit of independence, which must generally be broken before he can submit to be attended by the Parish Surgeon, which is usually followed by an apathy and indolence unfavourable to industry, and from which, reliance on parish pay is guaranteed for his family – and the workhouse for himself in his old age.'

The same argument as he had used in his petition to the House of Commons (but on that occasion couched in more temperate language). The comment about 'dealing wholesale with the bowels of the sick poor' would come back to haunt him; it was frequently flung at him by his opponents, most notably during the public 'spat' with the Coventry Charitable Dispensary in 1838.

He soldiered on, but would never offer a reason why he was for years the only surgeon at the Dispensary, and merely state that it was 'an affair too lengthy and too intricate to be explained here'. He remained resolutely discreet on the matter, but I sense much of it was of his own making.

However, he did not labour entirely alone; he employed a housekeeper in the Infirmary, and a dispenser ('Mr Walton') in the Dispensary, and, in due course, we know he had for various periods of time two assistants, Mr John Gardner MRCS and Mr Charles Nankivell MRCS, and also had an apprentice, Edward Bicknell, his brother-in-law:[41] together these two would establish

---

41   Edward (b. 1805), a younger brother of his wife, Mary. He also attended Guy's Hospital for the required six months of residence before taking the MRCS in 1830. After Southam, he then spent his entire career at the Self-Supporting Dispensary in Coventry.

the 'self-supporting dispensary' in Coventry, in 1831. He also had one or two, albeit short-lived, partnerships, so he wasn't completely ostracized by colleagues, even if most seemed to have kept their distance professionally.

The Second Annual Report of the Dispensary reveals that of 336 subscribers ('independent labourers and mechanics'), 270 – a high proportion – had used its services. The balance of subscriptions versus costs showed a surplus of £7 5s. 7d.

New subscribers from within six miles of the dispensary were encouraged, in the expectation that the proportion of subscribers actually making use of the Dispensary's services would fall, improving general finances.

Donations amounting to £22 18s. 6d. had been received in the previous year, and whilst gratefully acknowledged, the report reiterated that 'the Dispensary hopes to proceed independently of the Aid of the Rich in all its aspects'.

Dr John Conolly MD, who had been instrumental in setting up the dispensary in Stratford-upon-Avon in 1823, as mentioned earlier, joined the Committee of the Dispensary also.[42]

'Mr J T Gardner, surgeon, Southam', was present at the meeting as a 'Visitor'. John Turville Gardner MRCS 1824; LSA 1823, so in 1825 newly qualified, was for some years an assistant to Henry Lilley Smith. He was still working at the Dispensary during the cholera epidemic of 1832, but later left to practice in Brighton, at some indeterminate date.

Again there was an exhortation that 'all and every regular medical practitioner residing in the District can be admitted to the establishment at the discretion of the Committee'.

---

42   John Conolly, after his years at University College London, and subsequent return to Warwick, left Warwickshire again in 1839, to become Resident Physician at Middlesex County Asylum, where he abolished all forms of restraint of the mentally ill within three months of his arrival. The Warwick County Asylum at Hatton opened in 1852 and, under Dr Henry Parsey MD (a pupil of Conolly's), it too adopted a similar policy of non-restraint, to much commendation.

The provident dispensary movement gained momentum after Henry Lilley Smith's dispensary had opened, but the model for the other dispensaries following differed from Southam's; now three classes of patients were identified:

First Class: consisting of labourers or servants, if recommended by their master or mistress, earning less than £5 per annum and willing to subscribe for themselves.

Second Class: charity patients, not able to subscribe for themselves, but recommended by the Honorary Subscribers to the Dispensary, who could admit one patient for each half guinea subscribed, to a maximum of 1gn.

Third Class: parish paupers, unable to subscribe for themselves, but admitted by a contract for payment from the Overseers.

Funding was to come from the contributions of the First Class, the subscriptions of benevolent individuals for the Second Class, and sums paid by the parishes for their paupers, the Third Class.

Presumably, receiving 'the Aid of the Rich' for the Second Class of patients, which had been rejected in the initial Southam model, allowed the new dispensaries to have a more secure financial base, but in the event, the second class proved to be a financial drain on finances, in some cases insuperable, as we shall see.

Atherstone's dispensary opened in 1828, using a variation of the above model. Subscriptions from 'Honorary Members' and donations given were provided merely to supply cordials and linen, and pay nurses to attend the sick.

In its first year it provided for 765 subscribers: 'mechanics, servants and poor persons not receiving Parish Relief'. Paupers were admitted later. There were other modifications to Southam's system: the fee demanded was one penny a week for adults, and a ha'penny for children, 'patients to find their own bottles, bandages etc'.

Unlike Southam, midwifery was included – at a price: 'Any woman wishing to be attended in her confinement by a surgeon and paying eight shillings, before she is confined, may be attended by any one of the Dispensary Surgeons she might name.'

The Atherstone dispensary survived for only ten years: the town became very depressed economically following the end of the Napoleonic wars; its almost sole manufacturing base had been hat-making, and the demand for military caps evaporated almost overnight.

Henry Lilley Smith published and presented his ideas regarding this new model to a meeting of the 'London Society for Self-Supporting Charitable and Parochial Dispensaries', chaired by Lord Vernon at 32, Sackville Street, London on 20th March 1830. His main arguments were as before – that the security of medical care dispensaries provided for the labouring poor prevented them falling into pauperism and then might be removed by the Overseers to their own parishes, under the rules of settlement (discussed earlier), which was extremely disruptive to the persons involved, not to say expensive to the Parish. And the new system remunerated the doctors in a less objectionable manner – for the doctors – than competing for the annual contract of employment by the Vestry.

Provident dispensaries with a dispenser, he wrote, '… would reduce medical expenses by the lack of need for medicines to compound, day books to keep, bills to make out'.

Might this injure the income of the existing charitable societies, someone enquired? 'If so', he replied, 'so much the better. They may be made adjuncts to the prevention of cruelty to animals; under my scheme medical men would be paid for their skill, not requiring to gain their fees by medicines, as apothecaries do.' So there.

The campaign by doctors to be dignified by being paid for a consultation rather than merely for their medicines had been a lengthy one, and won only after a judgment in the High Court in January 1830. James Handey, a surgeon-apothecary in London, had submitted a bill of £7 0s. 6d. for 'medicines and attendance' (some fifteen visits) to a family by the name of Henson. Mr Henson refused to pay, claiming the cost of some twenty mixtures, pills, lotions and draughts was merely about £2 10s. 0d. Handey sued for payment of his bill in full. The jury decided in Handey's favour, and he was awarded damages of £7 0s. 6d. and costs.

There was delight at this ruling in Leamington, and at a meeting of local practitioners a resolution was proposed that '... the thanks of the medical profession are due to James Handey Esq of London for his exertions in obtaining the decision whereby the practitioner is entitled to be remunerated for his skill and time as well as for his medicines'.

Henry Lilley Smith (who was the Hon. Sec. of this society), also recorded the proposal '... that a subscription of 2/6d from each practitioner be raised immediately for the purpose of presenting Mr Handey with a piece of plate, and that the profession in London and throughout the country be invited to join the same'.

Establishing the principle was indeed a battle won, certainly, but it would take another thirty years before the war was finally won regarding its general acceptance.

According to the *Leamington Spa Courier*, his visit to the London Society was of 'little practical use and may be considered abortive' – this was because of some London medical men's distinct lack of interest in the scheme, coupled with a hostile anonymous letter to the Chairman (Henry Lilley Smith seemed to receive a number of these over the years, from more than one source).

His view of the matter was that, 'I struggled to be heard, where a third of the population, to whom Institutions of the like description would be a blessing: I explained to them they were neglecting a privilege and duty by not working with me.' As forthright as ever.

In fact, two attempts were made to form a London Society. The second also failed, but this time it was because the then Secretary of the Society absconded to Australia with the Society's funds (monies gathered from subscriptions and £200 – a considerable sum in 1831 – Henry Lilley Smith donated towards printing and publicity expenses).

Undeterred, the following year he published his proposal for 'establishing such a dispensary in every Market-Town and considerable Village in the Kingdom', in a pamphlet which included some very 'purple passages' of prose, for example:

> 'From these dispensaries many advantages will spring, and they will tend to unite the rich and the poor together in friendly relations and with a uniform bond of mutual regard as strongly as our Warwickshire blue lias cement does a church built of granite.'

As he wrote later, 'I [was] determined to become the centre of a great national movement on behalf of these dispensaries.' Ever singular of purpose, as we are well aware.

Whilst remaining the driving force almost single-handedly behind the day-to-day activities of both the Infirmary and Dispensary in Southam, Henry Lilley Smith was also involved in other philanthropic activities, mostly for the benefit of the town.

6

OTHER ACTIVITIES

What more does the monument outside the Infirmary tell the curious traveller? On the left-hand side of the monument is the inscription:

BOYS'
GARDEN ALLOTMENTS
FOR THEIR EARLY
INSTRUCTION IN THE
MANAGEMENT OF LAND
WERE ESTABLISHED HERE,
AND WERE VISITED
BY THE HONBle THE
SPEAKER OF THE
HOUSE OF COMMONS,
SIR JOHN FRANKLIN, THE
DOWAGER LADY NOEL BYRON
AND OTHERS

*

Allotments in Southam have existed since 1538, when 'Town Lands' were returned to the people ('common land') by Henry Vlll, some of which was divided into small half-acre plots with rents payable to the Rector and the Overseers of the Poor and administered as a charity, and which continue today on land on Welsh Road West. They have always been keenly sought after, providing as they do a source of food for the families of holders, the value of which being greatly in excess of rents charged. They were also viewed favourably in Victorian times, providing occupational therapy, encouraging thrift and self-sufficiency, and reducing opportunity for crime and drunkenness. And (in the eyes of the tenant), if a pig could be accommodated on the plot, so much the better.[43]

Henry Lilley Smith converted an acre of land near the dispensary on Warwick Road into allotments for schoolboys aged between eight and fourteen, who were chosen from a list given him by the headmaster of the National School in the town; this must have been a completely novel concept; usually only adults cultivated allotment plots. The boys were obliged to grow at least six kinds of vegetables, flowers, and herbs such as sage, mint, parsley, etc., and some even managed to cultivate fruit trees. No pigs were allowed.

Henry Lilley Smith was quoted as saying that establishing the allotments was 'less trouble than making arrangements for a charity ball'.

They attracted publicity; visitors included Sir John Franklin, a Royal Navy Officer and Arctic explorer, who later died whilst exploring the North West Passage in 1845, and Lady Noel Byron, widow of the poet Lord Byron.[44]

---

43   A pig ('The gentleman who pays the rent') would provide sufficient (cured) pork for a family for the best part of a winter.

44   Byron's widow established in 1858 the 'Lady Noel Byron Nursing Association Fund' for the provision of a district nurse for the villages of East and West Horsley, in Surrey; she also made a donation to the Henry Lilley Smith Memorial Fund in 1859.

Why such widespread interest was shown in these allotments must have been purely due to their novelty.

The allotments continued for about ten years, giving the boys practical experience of 'land husbandry' and elementary botany, whilst producing food for their families. A small library of some sixty books was also kept in Henry Lilley Smith's house for the boys; these were, he said, for the most part, 'donations from the nurseries of the rich to the families of the poor'.

'In the year 1824, the late Mr Thomas Bicknell [his wife's father] and others were induced to divide 50 acres amongst the labourers and mechanics of Southam, the effect of which proved highly beneficial.' Further allotments were started in 1832, this time in nearby Harbury, on land that Henry Lilley Smith had partly inherited from his maternal grandfather Henry Chambers, and partly purchased himself. The sixty allotments were from half an acre to an acre in size; they must have taken a lot of tending, given that cultivating the soil was limited to 'spade husbandry', and most allotments could only be worked on in the evenings and at weekends, and not at all on Sundays. In addition to the usual vegetable crops, here the tenants were encouraged to keep a pig (unlike Southam), which improved the family's diet immeasurably. In fact, the loss of a pig would prove a severe dietary loss to the family and a financial blow to the owner. Later in the century, the Southam Pig Club (founded in 1878) and the Burton Dassett Pig Society (founded in 1886) – there were others – were formed to provide owners with insurance against such a loss.

Whilst administering the Harbury allotments, he also had the idea of forming the Harbury Sick Club (or 'Alfred Friendly Society'), a small club of about twenty members, managed by himself and two collectors, thereby making a committee – in his view – 'unnecessary'.[45] For a weekly donation of 3d. each member would be insured for 6s./week for up to seven weeks in any one year, if disabled by accident or sickness. On the death of a member, one shilling was subscribed by all the members towards his funeral expenses (minimum £2 10s. 0d.); and if his wife died, 6d. was paid by each member (minimum £1 10s. 0d.) to the surviving spouse.

The attitude to charity was hardening with the introduction of the New Poor Laws, and becoming very selective. The Poor Laws and the workhouse provided for the aged, infirm, insane (up to a point), foundlings and unwed mothers; charities were to provide support in the form of hospitals and dispensaries for those who were ill by no fault of their own. Did 'sick clubs' help? Again, up to a point: they did not, in the main, accept women or children, nor those whose trade or occupation incurred a degree of substantial risk of injury or death, for example, knife sharpeners, thatchers or needlegrinders (who frequently sustained eye injuries and tended to die prematurely from 'pointer's rot' – lung disease from inhaled metal dust).

So the Alfred Friendly Society was an improvement for Harbury's populace, at least.

Henry Lilley Smith's intention was 'to establish as many Alfred Societies as possible in each parish', but such a grandiose proposal didn't really get off the ground, despite the wider publicity of a pamphlet which he published in 1837 aimed at 'the governors and free members of self-supporting dispensaries and penny clubs', in which he wrote 'my object is to make "*a paradise of old England*"' [his italics] and concluded 'that there can be no order, harmony, and unity in the world unless it is based on Divine precepts of government'. No such thing as a free lunch. Perhaps these sentiments diluted enthusiasm.

---

45   Named after King Alfred the Great, who had encouraged local responsibility by dividing the Kingdom into 'shires', 'hundreds' and 'tythings' – much like the counties, districts and parishes of today.

Henry Lilley Smith seemed to perpetually rub people's fur up the wrong way. The tone of another article he wrote in 1842 regarding the Harbury Sick Club suggests why, when he discusses how the labourer's life would be improved by the scheme:

'By these means, some spirit, life, and good feeling would be instilled into and encouraged to abide with us, despite the Mammons and Molochs that haunt and infest society – who would probably smell their way to the Guardians' [of the Poor] committee room as naturally as bats and goblins do to dark and cheerless places.'

Local landowners and clergy were somewhat proprietorial in their attitude towards 'their' workers and parishioners and found his egalitarian attitude misplaced and benevolence towards the poor threatening and I sense they also found such intemperate language difficult to accept.

Anyway, it was too much. After the allotments had been in existence for a number of years, persons unknown – but thought to be local farmers – presumably considered that the local workforce working on the land to provide for themselves allowed them far too much independence. The allotments were damaged and destroyed. The perpetrators were never discovered.

*

The cholera epidemic of 1832 and 'The Southam Cholera Assurance Society'

In 1832, cholera became epidemic in England: by August, 22,960 cases and 8,595 deaths had been reported. It got worse before it got better.[46] If infection was severe, death from dehydration would occur rapidly, coming soon after the onset of symptoms of diarrhoea and vomiting; a common remedy advised was to drink 'half a pint of warm water in which as much common salt as possible has been dissolved and then to take 25 drops of laudanum [opium] in a small glass of any agreeable drink'. A reasonable enough approach to attempt to replace fluid loss and control diarrhoea ordinarily, but for cholera it proved ineffectual.

Henry Lilley Smith and the Rector of Southam, Revd Charles Bathurst, established 'The Southam Cholera Assurance Society', to form a fund 'for maintenance in sickness, for funeral expenses, and for a gratuity to widows, widowers, and children who may be deprived of parents by the cholera'.

How did it work? 'Any head of a family subscribing from 3d. to 5s. weekly will be allowed twelve times the amount of his subscription daily when any of his family are attacked with cholera, to the time of recovery or death. Any person subscribing from 3d. to 1s. weekly, will be allowed £3 in case of death of a parent. For a servant or child of a subscriber who shall die of cholera, £2 shall be allowed. The subscriptions to be continued until the cholera has ceased for twenty miles round Southam; and when no further cause for apprehension exists of the disease breaking out in Southam, each subscriber is to receive back his subscription.'

How did Southam fare in the epidemic? Not too badly, all considered. Henry Lilley Smith gave an account of the 1832 cholera outbreak in Southam, and some advice on treatment (as he saw it), in a letter to the *Provincial Medical and Surgical Journal*, dated 20th May 1849 (when there was a further epidemic of cholera in the country):

---

46   In 1842, the Poor Law Commissioner Edwin Chadwick published his 'Report on the Sanitary Conditions of the Labouring People'. It was grim reading; some 16,000 people in total had died in the 1832 epidemic. In 1847, a Public Health Bill was defeated in the House of Commons, MPs balking at the cost required to implement it, allegedly. A fresh epidemic in 1848 caused it to be passed in the Commons – with some alacrity.

'Cholera was introduced twice; once into the town and once into a village, by a boatman's family, about two miles from us, and three persons lost their lives, although it never extended from the place it was brought. I attribute this checking of its course mainly to the public confidence the "Cholera Assurance Society" gave to the medical men, and for submitting to having those things done for them good naturedly, which I am sure they would have at least grumbled at if it had been done by Act of Parliament.

For instance, when a case of cholera was reported to us, I went with Mr Gardner (now of Brighton), and we caused the door of the cottage (a barber and tripe-dresser's), to be surrounded by hurdles, and gave strict orders to have no person, except the doctors and nurses, to visit the house. We also ordered a fire of shavings etc. to be kept burning before the door, within the fence, for we thought it good sense to rarify the atmosphere before the door and so dilute and carry away anything offensive upwards. It succeeded, for though the patient died, there was no extension of the disease.[47]

It may be encouraging to add, that by placing the money in the Savings Bank, as it was paid in weekly, and by allowing the interest to accumulate, with the aid of a donation, we were enabled, some months afterwards, to restore to each of the subscribers the entire amount of his accumulated payments.'

Henry Lilley Smith's ability to rub people's fur up the wrong way appears to have increased with age; the final paragraph to the above letter is startling:

---

47   The connection between cholera infection and contaminated water by 'excramental distribution' was only made by Dr John Snow in 1856, when new cases ceased after he removed the pump handle to a public well in Broad Street in Soho, London, which was dispensing contaminated water. The identification of the bacterial cause, *Vibrio cholerae*, was made in 1884 by the German microbiologist, Robert Koch.

'I have also sent you [the editor of the Journal] an address to the labourers etc., [now lost] which was eagerly purchased, and, proceeding from a medical man who was known to them, I think had more influence over them than any dry official papers from a remote Board of Health could be expected to have. I am afraid it is too long for insertion in your Journal, but something of the kind issued by the local friends of the people, would be more useful than anything likely to come from the great Crowned image of Somerset House, whose little toe of iron and miry clay, at Southam, would trample on any man who should seek to improve the condition of the honestly independent labourer.'

Not easy to fathom, but this was probably a passing reference to the recent 1848 Removal of Nuisances Act, prompted by the repeated cholera epidemics, which provided a legal mechanism involving medical certification and orders from the Justices of the Peace 'for the speedy removal of certain nuisances [unspecified] and the prevention of contagious and epidemic diseases'. It might also have been used (but this is only supposition) regarding pigs on allotments – the keeping of pigs was often a cause for complaint by other residents; in Leamington many properties in the old town also had pigsties behind them, and sanitation was rudimentary.

It was a reasonable sentiment on Henry Lilley Smith's part, but the language used is 'robust', to say the least.

One can easily hear him uttering those words, if one looks at the portrait photograph, taken in his later years, with his shock of white hair and pugnacious expression reminiscent of a bad-tempered Jack Russell terrier. Quite a force to be reckoned with, in any argument, is my impression – one can almost hear him say "We are not debating this matter; I am right, and you are wrong" – and doubtless he was a difficult colleague to work with, notwithstanding the many comments about his 'earnest philanthropy'. Too earnest, perhaps.

*

Continuing the circuit of the monument, the following inscription can be found on its right-hand side:

THE POPULAR
DISPENSARY
MAYPOLE HOLIDAY
WAS HELD HERE
TO THE ENJOYMENT
OF THE INHABITANTS
OF THIS TOWN
FOR MANY YEARS

*

'Here flow'ry garlands were entwined
The lofty pole to grace
And MAY had all her charms combined
To decorate the place'

*

The Maypole Holiday

What was 'The Popular Dispensary Maypole Holiday'?

Southam had held a 'Show Fair', or the 'Godiva Procession', an ancient, possibly a fertility (of the land), festival held on the first Monday in June, which by the 1800s had become 'a drunken bacchanalia'. In Henry Lilley Smith's opinion: '... it had attracted to its pleasures, the young and gay of both sexes, as well as the vicious and dissipated of all grades, from a circuit of many miles in extent [...] but all attempts to suppress it had proved in vain; at the best of times it was an abominable affair.'

However, he decided to lie low and bide his time: 'The experience I had obtained when first establishing the Infirmary and Dispensary induced for me in the future to be more cautious in my attempts to carry out annihilation of this revolting exhibition.'

But, in the fullness of time, annihilated it was. His plan was to erect a maypole on the land behind his house 'for an annual fête, to be known as the Southam Dispensary Spring Holiday' and 'invite to the celebration of its attendant rustic games, the members, wives and children of the self-supporting Dispensary, with the view to making it a general holiday and an innocent source of recreation to young persons of all classes, from all the country round'. This proved very successful, for he wrote later, 'soon after the *second* [his italics] anniversary of our rural fête, the show fair was given up, never again, I trust, to be revived'.

What went on in the new fête, that it should have been so successful in replacing the Show Fair (which sounds to have been rather fun)?

Limiting the entrants, apart from the Free Members and their families, by ticket of admission, and controlling the crowds, for the main part by allowing into the fête no liquors or spirits, but 'such an allowance of good fresh beer, with bread and cheese, is permitted as will do a man good', seems to have been the lynchpin.[48]

Southam Heritage has a ticket of admission for the tenth Dispensary Spring Holiday, on Thursday 21st May 1835, in its archive – on the reverse of which is printed:

---

48   No puritan he, perhaps, despite our suspicions? But one moment: a footnote to his 1842 description of the Maypole Holiday lowers the spirits somewhat – it states solemnly: 'tea is now substituted'. His temperament plainly allowed him to contribute towards the gaiety of nations – but only up to a point...

'The principal object of this Dispensary is to provide, by a Mutual Association, against the Expenses of Sickness, by carrying into practical execution the command to "bear one another's burdens"; – a secondary object is to promote that cordial union and friendly intercourse which ought to exist amongst neighbours, and by bringing together with their families, for some innocent recreation occasionally, make a manifest distinction between the comparatively improvident, – between those who do what they can for their families, and those who do nothing but exhaust the money in Bridewell, Jails, or Workhouses, which would otherwise be paid for labour.

The party will break up at 9 o'clock and it is expected the Free Members will not loiter in the town, or adjourn to the Public Houses, but leave at the same time with their families and go home together. God Save the King and Rule, Britannia, as usual, at parting.'

Difficult to maintain a head of steam of jollification all afternoon, after reading that, I would have thought.

A report in the *Leamington Spa Courier* of 16th May 1829 gives some idea of the character of the fête:

'The Members of the Self-supporting Dispensary assembled on Wednesday the 13th instant, to spend the surplus funds accumulated by the Institution during the past year – According to annual custom, this scene of rural festivity occurred in a field situated at the back of Mr Smith's house, where was placed a May-pole about 50 feet in height, surmounted by the device of an Imperial Crown, and decorated with ribbons, comprising all the colours of the rainbow; garlands, woven with great taste and contributed by the ladies of the town and neighbourhood, being tastefully suspended from it under the able direction of an appointed manager [...]. The extremity of the Green, which was appropriated to the use of the ladies, was tastefully decorated with wreaths of laurel, oak, flowers, and garlands.

At about four o'clock the Free Members to the Dispensary proceeded to the Craven Arms, where they partook of beef and pudding, and a quart of ale each man. The wives and children of the Members about the same hour partook of a grateful repast, consisting of tea and cake under the tent.

At five o'clock the Members returned again to the Green, which about that time was thronged by the principal inhabitants of the town and surrounding villages, and the Military Brass Band, from Leamington, played some lively and popular airs at intervals during the evening.

Dancing was continued with unremitting activity until the evening's amusements were concluded by the company forming themselves into a large circle, and the whole party enthusiastically singing in full chorus the National Anthem of God Save the King. We have great pleasure in adding that the Free Members returned to their homes in the greatest decorum; without evincing any of those imprudent and intemperate acts which are too frequently apt to occur when fathers of families do not consider their wives and children as primary objects of attention. The scene we witnessed on this occasion speaks volumes in favour of the Self-Supporting Dispensary system.'

So, Henry Lilley Smith, by sheer force of personality, socially engineered for Southam an afternoon of 'cordial union and friendly intercourse', which terminated with the National Anthem before dispersal; unlike the end of the Show Fair, when, much to his disapproval, '... males and females, after figuring in the spectacle during the day, contrived to affright the town from its propriety by night, and enact in its streets, scenes of every kind of vice – drunkenness, profaneness, and prostitution.'

But he may have underestimated the resilience of Southam's residents; when Joseph Ashby visited the town in 1880 he was struck by 'the great number of public houses, out of all proportion to the size of the town.'[49]

The Maypole Holiday was unrelated to the ancient 'Mop Fair', the annual hiring fair in the town, when labourers and servants offered themselves for work, and – with luck – were hired by prospective employers for the coming twelve months (minus a day), and then celebrated by hitting the local public houses in the evening. The Maypole Holiday (such as it was) for the town may be long lost, but the 'Mop' continues, on the Monday afternoon and evening in October nearest to Michaelmas Day. Today, it is organised by Southam Lions, and is merely a pig roast for charity in the afternoon and a fun-fair which carries on into the evening, and which is dismantled at its close and long departed by the following morning.

Henry Lilley Smith had other, wider political and philanthropic interests.

*

Provincial Medical and Surgical Association

Dr Charles Hastings, a physician at Worcester Infirmary, on 18th July 1832, arranged a meeting of over fifty doctors from all over the United Kingdom, apart from London, in the boardroom of the hospital with the intention of forming 'an Association for the friendly sharing of scientific knowledge between doctors.'

---

49   Joseph Ashby (1859–1919); born in Tysoe, he was an agricultural trades unionist and advocate of Friendly Societies for self-help.

This proved surprisingly popular at a time when most doctors outside hospital worked in isolation, and usually in competition for patients.

It eventually admitted London doctors as members in 1853 and in 1856 became the British Medical Association.

Dr John Conolly, then back in practice in Warwick after his unhappy time in London, was among those doctors present in the boardroom for that meeting; Henry Lilley Smith was one of the 266 inaugural members, but was 'regrettably detained by paramount necessity' from being present in person in Worcester – as were a number of other local physicians and surgeons, including Dr Henry Jephson of Leamington and Mr Henry Blenkinsop, surgeon to the Warwick Dispensary and the County Gaol. All remained members for the rest of their careers.

*

Shoeblack Brigades

Henry Lilley Smith was one of the early proponents of Shoeblack Brigades, according to the obituary in the *Leamington Spa Courier*. This concept of 'providing work of an honest but low kind' was first formulated in 1850 by three teachers at the Ragged School in London (which provided lodging and a basic education for destitute and orphaned children, who were often debarred from Sunday Schools by virtue of their appearance or unruly behaviour).

Boys from age twelve or fourteen were kitted out in red jackets and black aprons and with a shoebox were given a pitch on a street in London's West End, allocated by the police who rotated pitches twice a week (some being more lucrative than others). Each customer paid a flat rate of one penny to have their shoes cleaned; and with the volume of horse-drawn traffic in London at the time, there was probably good reason.

Of their daily income, one third went on their keep in a hostel, one third into a savings account in their name and one third was returned to the boy. At age eighteen, a boy was then found a 'suitable position' as a servant or apprentice, or went to sea, or emigrated to America – presumably as an indentured servant. ('Indentured servants' had their cost of passage paid by their future employer in return for a number of years – usually seven – spent as a servant or in unpaid agricultural labour, often with pretty harsh treatment. It was, in essence, close to slavery, but a very convenient method of removing – for better or worse – various social undesirables.)

The Brigades, each with their own distinctive uniforms, proved very successful and could be found in London, and other large cities, well into the twentieth century.

7

ESTABLISHED PRACTICE

Henry Lilley Smith may not have been a pillar of the church – he doesn't appear to have been a churchwarden or similar – but he seems to have been something of a pillar of the community, and not just merely as an expression of his status in the town as a medical man: at midday on 9th September 1831 (the day after the Coronation of William IV), a Coronation dinner was held on Market Hill, for which subscriptions had been invited 'to defray the expense regarding the poor inhabitants of the Town'. Sixty-six subscriptions were received, totalling £42 5s 0d: Henry donated 2 gns (no one donated more than he), 'Mrs Smith' donated 10s, and his father, W L Smith, donated 1gn.

The dinner made a profit of £5 2s 5d, after expenses (which included '£1 0s 0d to bell ringers').

Inside the small book of the accounts for the dinner there is tucked a ticket for a seat at the 'Victoria Coronation Dinner' in 1838 at Daventry, which states: 'each person to bring a knife, fork, plate and mug'. One hopes it did not become too rowdy later on.

Some years later there was another appeal for funds: this time it was Queen Victoria's letter of January 1847 to her subjects, urging them to donate towards the provision of aid for the sufferers of the Irish famine. The Smith family donated handsomely (and again none more so than they): Henry Lilley Smith donated £3; Mrs H L Smith donated £2; 'Miss Sophy Smith' donated 10/-; 'Mrs Smith (sen)' donated £2; and 'Green (infirmary)' a modest 6d. He was possibly an inpatient. £77 9s 6d was collected by the town (out of a national total of £170,571).

Curiously no other doctors in the town appear in either of the subscription lists.

Henry Lilley Smith became a freemason in 1835: was it the philanthropic element of masonry which attracted him, or was it a more personal interest? He was admitted a Freeman of Lodge 556 (Leamington Priors), to join fellow masons Henry Jephson, Charles Loudon, John Pritchard, Thomas Hewlett and Amos Middleton: all local physicians and surgeons, distinguished in their fields, and a sure sign of his acceptance into established medical practice in the county.

This might suggest that progress in a medical career in the years after the Napoleonic wars was fairly painless, but that was not the case. Careers could be fragile (unlike today, when a medical degree, some hard work acquiring post-graduate degrees and diplomas – and a bit of luck at interview – offers a stable and long-term career within the NHS); then, competition to make an adequate living was fierce, especially with a large influx of medical men from the army and navy (with varying degrees of medical and surgical training) seeking practice vacancies or just merely 'putting up one's plate' and awaiting patients to darken the door: it was said in 1842 that 'by the time when a physician earns his bread and cheese he has no longer the teeth to eat them with.'

Inevitably there were some failures, as the following item from the *London Gazette* (where all bankruptcies had to be reported) identifies:

'Warwick Courthouse 2nd December 1837

Richard Lea, heretofore lodging at Thomas Court's, the Unicorn Inn in the West-Street, Warwick, out of business, then of Wellesbourne, Surgeon, but now a prisoner in the Gaol of Warwick, for debt.'

Exactly what occasioned Richard Lea's Hogarthian 'Rake's Progress' has not been ascertainable; of course, it may well have been due to any number of causes, be they circumstantial, ill health, profligacy, or even the slippery slope to ruin occasioned by 'the demon drink', so graphically illustrated some ten years later by George Cruikshank (son of Isaac Cruikshank of 'A Vestry Dinner' fame) in his series of etchings 'The Bottle'; yet again one can only surmise, perhaps silently give thanks, and quickly move on to other matters.

By the mid-1840s, both the Infirmary and the Dispensary had been in existence for over twenty years, and some twenty other eye (and ear) infirmaries were also in existence, scattered around the country; the closest being Birmingham Eye Hospital, which had opened in 1824.

Although some provident dispensaries, such as Atherstone, had failed in the early years after 1823, a number were established successfully – in Coventry, Derby, Lymington (Hants) in 1831, and the Royal Victoria Dispensary, Northampton in 1845 ; in London Marylebone (Charlotte Street) opened in 1833, Paddington (Start Street) in 1838, St John's Wood (Henstridge Villas) in 1844 and Hampstead (New End) in 1845: there were others.

Leamington Spa was a notable latecomer, in 1869, to the movement. This was probably because there were a number of establishments already in existence which provided medical aid to the poor: Benjamin Satchwell had established his 'Leamington Spa Charity' in 1806, which provided medicinal saline baths to the sick poor at 'Abbott's Original Baths' (demolished in 1867);

a charitable infirmary (with ten beds) with a dispensary had also been established in 1824 on the corner of Regent Street and Bedford Street (the site of an earlier dispensary built in 1816 by Dr Amos Middleton, adjacent to his private residence, Belsay House, in Bedford Street).[50] Henry Lilley Smith was appointed 'Oculist' (but not 'Aurist') to this new infirmary, a year younger than Southam's.

It would be replaced, in its turn, in 1834, by a new hospital with fifty beds in Radford Road, known as 'The Warneford General Bathing Institution & Leamington Hospital', with Dr Amos Middleton as its attending physician; it was so titled because it incorporated Benjamin Satchwell's charity for the practice of prescribing saline baths.[51] Henry Lilley Smith was not appointed 'Oculist' to the new hospital, but the Southam Eye & Ear Infirmary was a generous subscriber of 50 gns *per annum*, which gave him rights to a substantial number of inpatient and outpatient 'tickets'.

So, it was not until after Henry Lilley Smith's death that a provident dispensary would open in a fine Regency house in Holly Walk, in 1869. It seems to me it was more than possible that Leamington's physicians waited until there was absolutely no possibility that Henry Lilley Smith would become, or try to become, influential in running it.

Not as many dispensaries throughout the land as Henry Lilley Smith might have wished, perhaps; their long-term success seems only to have been due to a radical re-appraisal of the original policy

---

50   Belsay House was named after Belsay Castle, the Middleton family home in Northumberland. The Leamington Tennis Court Club was built to the other side of it in 1846, described by the *Leamington Spa Courier* as 'a splendid specimen of Batchelors' Hall'. Women would eventually be accepted as members in 2011.

51   The hospital came to be known as 'The Warneford Hospital' in recognition of the substantial sums of money gifted to it by the Revd Samuel Warneford, an eccentric benefactor who had himself previously attended the Pump Room baths; the Radcliffe Lunatic Asylum, Oxford, was likewise renamed 'The Warneford Hospital, Oxford' in 1843, for the same reason.

regarding the patients they were to provide for. In many cases, the numbers of 'Second Class' (charity) patients seen and treated had been greatly in excess of those of the 'First Class' (fee-paying). Many of the 'Second Class' appeared to be capable of being, but somehow were reluctant to be, 'First Class' subscribers; other 'Second Class' patients appeared to be well within the fee-paying subscriber class as regards annual income, yet managed to obtain charity tickets of admission, given indiscriminately by some charitable subscribers, a practice which was much deplored but difficult to prevent. Henry Lilley Smith had had the same problem with admissions to his Infirmary. In the event, many provident dispensaries decided to provide their services merely to the fee-paying class.

Henry Lilley Smith wrote to John Jones, the surgeon to the Derby Dispensary in 1841:

'When I first proposed to establish a charity class of patients in conjunction with the self-supporting and parochial, it was for this town (Southam) when at the time we had no Dispensary or Infirmary whatever, indeed, there was none near us. I was soon obliged to abandon the charity class, for the simple fact that *the poor would not pay for themselves as long as anybody would pay for them* [his italics].

The same was the case at Wellesburn [sic], at Atherstone, at Nuneaton, all places where the self-supporting cases would have done well, had it not been for the indiscreet recommendations into the '"charity class".' [All three closed after about ten years in existence.] I, therefore, long ago advised at Coventry and other places, a Dispensary on the self-supporting principle *alone,* and they would have worked well.

As you have a General Hospital [with a charitable dispensary] at Derby, there can be less harm in throwing the "charity class" overboard.'

Intimations of this decision can be detected in that the Infirmary accepted admissions from charitable subscribers, but when it came to establish the Dispensary some five years on, it did not.

Regarding the paupers, however, the provision of social welfare in England had changed with the Poor Law Amendment Act of 1834; care by each parish was replaced by about 2,500 'Unions', each amalgamating a number of parishes: this made their care, under what was to be known as the 'New Poor Law', much less costly in terms of medical manpower, but almost invariably meant admission to the 'workhouse' – 'indoor relief' as it was termed. For the most part this came to replace 'out relief' – the old method of providing care and financial support to destitute families in their homes by the parish.

This letter, from 'a retired naval surgeon', was published in *The Lancet* on 20th October 1836:

'The Board of Governors wish to appoint a duly qualified surgeon who will devote his full time to the duties of Medical Officer to Leighton Buzzard Union Parishes (a total of 11,800 persons), providing due and punctual attendance in all medical, surgical and midwifery cases and will provide all medicines, drugs and medical and surgical requisites (trusses excepted). Unfurnished accommodation and stable-room will be provided. Annual salary £200.

Compare this to a Naval surgeon. A ship-of-war and crew numbers 900 persons, therefore thirteen such ships will number 11,700. All medicines are provided by the Government. Every ship has one Surgeon and three assistant surgeons, board and lodging provided. A Surgeon's annual pay is £159 9s. 4d., an assistant's £119 12s. 0d. Total pay = £6,737 9s. 4d. for a population of 100 less than Leighton Buzzard Union.

Pay for Army Surgeons is comparable: and there is an allowance for the keep of a horse.

I have often wished that Parish Surgeons were appointed and paid by the Government.'

One can understand why in 1810 William Dent (with his interest in horses), had so swiftly decided on a military career.

The Parish Overseers, now known as 'Guardians of the Poor', persisted with the administrative mechanism of 'farming out' medical care by annual contract until 1842, when it was abolished, the Poor Law Commissioners determining '… competition should turn on the [medical men's] respective character and skills, not on the sum at which they may be severally willing to undertake the office'.

Be that as it may, many Guardians continued to administer their Unions as they always had done. Henry Lilley Smith would berate the Guardians' parsimonious behaviour regularly in his annual reports, especially their tardiness in settling accounts (if indeed they ever paid at all) for fees for parish patients attending the Dispensary or Infirmary under contracts drawn up with the various Guardians.

Southam's original 'poorhouse', built in the early 1700s for the parish, was capable of housing up to twenty aged or infirm inmates, but held only ten when Henry Lilley Smith returned to Southam in 1811; in 1837, under the New Poor Law, a considerably larger workhouse on Welsh Road West was built to house about eighty inmates, for the new catchment area or 'Union', an amalgamation of some seventeen local parishes, replacing the small poorhouses at Southam, Napton and Grandborough. Inmates were given free lodging and the most basic of food and sustenance, in exchange for manual labour of one type or another. The Unions soon found they were dealing with the elderly, the infirm, children and occasionally the insane (being very much cheaper than occupying a bed in an asylum). Families were strictly segregated by sex and age; it was not an institution one would care to enter, unless there was absolutely no alternative. But that was the object.

The workhouse was converted to (very inadequate) housing in 1923, known as 'The Dwellings', which was eventually demolished in the 1960s – to much general rejoicing in the town. Southam Primary School now stands on the site.

In Coventry, there had been something of a public spat between supporters of the new provident dispensary, established in 1831 with some success (by 1833 it had 2,500 subscribers), in spite of what Henry Lilley Smith's son, William, described some years later in a letter to the BMJ as 'considerable opposition and the prejudiced dislike of some of his profession', who were supporters of the charitable dispensary which had been in existence there since about 1793.

The spat was carried out through the medium of the correspondence columns of the *Leamington Spa Courier* and the *Coventry Herald* newspapers, where Mr Charles Nankivell, previously Henry Lilley Smith's assistant in Southam and by then one of the two medical officers at Coventry, argued that early presentation at the provident dispensary meant that a successful outcome for any episode of illness was higher than in charitable dispensaries, where presentation was subject to delay by the need to obtain a ticket of attendance: 'in Coventry, of 6,094 Provident patients 92 had died – 1 in 66. At Chorlton-on-Medlock [a Manchester suburb], in the same period, of 6,438 Charitable patients, 210 had died – 1 in 30.'

Eventually the two institutions came to an uneasy truce; the provident dispensary continued its activities from Bayley Lane, on the one hand, in premises opposite the churchyard of the medieval St Michael's Church[52] and the charitable dispensary's continued survival was aided by its combining with the new

---

52   From 1918 onwards, Coventry's Cathedral; it was destroyed by the Luftwaffe on 14th November 1940, during World War II, and replaced by the new cathedral, built adjacent to its ruins.

hospital (of one ward and fourteen beds) in 1840 in a building purchased in Little Park Street.

The need for a hospital in Coventry was plainly pressing; the editor of the *Coventry Herald* had written in 1838:

'It is high time that the poor of the City had some other refuge than the workhouse in time of sickness. The old corporators annually swallowed in hock, champagne and venison, as much of the public charities as would have supported a hospital.'

So, Cruikshank's 1795 cartoon of the behaviour of the Vestry plainly had much more than just a mere grain of truth in it.

The newspaper's campaign proved successful: the charitable dispensary moved into a fine purpose-built building in 1864 – the Coventry & Warwickshire Hospital, Stony Stanton Lane.[53]

As we know, Henry Lilley Smith was responsible for the Infirmary and the Dispensary single-handed for almost his whole career, despite his exhortations to other medical men to join him. Of those who did become involved, for some reason or other, their professional relationships were short-lived.

He had employed assistants in the Dispensary from time to time; Charles Nankivell from 1829–1831, and Edward Bicknell, who had been his apprentice, both went to open the Coventry Dispensary; John Gardner had assisted him for some years, and during the 1832 cholera epidemic, before moving to Brighton, and in 1841 a 'George Sherard, aged 15' appears on the census form as lodger in the cottage next to the Infirmary, and is described as 'surgeon's apprentice' but no further trace of him can be found.[54]

At about this time, for a few years, Henry Lilley Smith was

53 The Coventry & Warwickshire Hospital closed with the opening of Walsgrave Hospital (later University Hospital).

54 George Sherard does not appear in the records of Licentiates of the Society of Apothecaries, nor Members of the Royal College of Surgeons of England, nor the Medical Register (from 1859).

in a most unlikely partnership with Charles Cowdell, who was in practice in Oundle, some miles east of Northampton, as 'oculists, aurists, surgeons and apothecaries under the firm of Cowdell and Smith'. Dr Charles Cowdell (not to be confused with George Lowdell) had qualified MRCS, LSA in 1837, and appears to have begun practice in New Street, Oundle, in about 1841. The partnership was 'dissolved' in 1843, so Henry Lilley Smith can only have been in partnership with him for some two years. It seems extraordinary to attempt to sustain a medical partnership at that distance in the 1840s, especially given travelling conditions. I suspect Charles Cowdell merely came to Northampton to assist with the outpatient clinics held there. After marrying in 1842, he left Oundle in 1849 for the position of physician to the Dorset County Infirmary in Dorchester, where he ended his career.

Interestingly, in 1848 he wrote a paper on cholera with the unwieldy title *A Disquisition on Pestilential Cholera (an attempt to explain its phenomena, nature, cause, prevention and treatment by reference to its extrinsic fungal origin)* – in which he proposed (erroneously) a fungus, much like yeast, as cause, it being inhaled into the lungs and thence into the blood stream. As to treatment, he advised a facemask made from cloth impregnated with oil of cloves – shades of the Venetian physicians wearing beaky masks stuffed with herbs as a filter of the air whilst treating plague victims – but in essence, this was merely a variation on the prevailing view that the disease was a 'miasma' (air-borne); hence Henry Lilley Smith's burning of bonfires outside the houses of those infected with cholera, 'to dilute and carry away anything offensive upwards'.

Later, John Burt MD (Edinburgh) was briefly his partner from about 1845–1848, until that partnership was also terminated, this time 'by mutual consent', but for reasons unknown. John Burt's entry in the 1865 Medical Directory states he had been 'late physician to Hunningham Lunatic Asylum and Southam Eye and

Ear Infirmary'.[55] In 1862 he turns up in practice in Harwich, is a JP, and 'physician to the Dovercourt Spa'.[56]

*

There were a surprising number of other medical men in Southam in the first half of the 1800s, given its size – it is a wonder it could support so many.

George Lowdell, his presumed competitor for the post of Parish Surgeon in 1811, was joined in practice in partnership a few years later by Wright Laxton of Marholm, Peterborough, who had qualified LSA in 1816, then married Alice Dean from nearby Longthorpe in August 1817, and who came to Southam in 1818, where he rented a tenement from George Cooke of Stoneythorpe. George Lowdell and he practised together as 'Surgeons and Apothecaries' in the town until their partnership was dissolved 'by mutual agreement' in 1823, whereupon George Lowdell moved to Brighton.

The first of George and Jessamine Lowdell's four sons (also named George) had been born in Southam on 22nd November 1813 (and probably others of their twelve children too). George junior became MRCS in 1835 and was later appointed surgeon to the (now Royal) Sussex County Hospital in Brighton. His father remained in practice in Brighton until his retirement.

Wright Laxton stayed on in practice in Southam for some years: in 1828 he is recorded as living in 'Tomwell House, Southam', with his wife Alice and four sons; Alice died

---

55   Hunningham House was a private asylum in Harbury accommodating seventy patients, which closed when the County Asylum at Hatton opened in 1852.

56   Dovercourt, a seaside resort near Harwich, opened a spa in 1852, claiming 'the waters are in great repute, possessing medicinal properties similar to the waters of Tunbridge Wells'. It was closed down during WW1; the local Medical Officer of Health, seemingly, was unimpressed by the quality of the waters.

prematurely, aged thirty-eight, and was buried in St James's churchyard in February 1834. By 1838 he too had moved away to practise as a 'surgeon and farmer' in Littleport, Cambridgeshire, and was remarried, this time to Ellen Earl, a Marholm girl some ten years his junior.

Edward Welchman was to become one of the longest established doctors in the town: he came from a medical family (almost all the male members of which confusingly appear to have been christened Edward) who for over a century had been successively surgeons in Kineton, the small market town very similar in size to Southam, about nine miles distant. Firstly, John Welchman (1729–1799) had been in practice there; secondly, his son Edward Sr. (1756–1831); thirdly, Edward Jr. (1789–1845) and lastly, Southam's Edward (1814–1865), whose son – also Edward – kicked over the traces and became a farmer at Ufton.

Southam's Edward Welchman, after qualifying MRCS, LSA in 1837, with the Silver Medal in Anatomy in 1833 from the new Birmingham School of Medicine, set up in practice in Wood Street, where he was to outlive Henry Lilley Smith; he would be joined in practice in 1860 by a young bachelor surgeon, Thomas Edward Ruttledge – his father also being Thomas Ruttledge, he was known as Edward – who, after training at the London Hospital, qualified MRCS in 1857. In the three years before he arrived in Southam he had also gained the LM (Licentiate in Midwifery) diploma from the Rotunda Hospital, Dublin – thus becoming the first contemporary of Henry Lilley Smith in the Southam area to profess a special interest (and proficiency, one would expect) in the subject. Perhaps this reflects a conscientious personality.

*

Now it gets a little complicated: John Montgomery (b. 1791), an Aberdonian physician (with an MD from Glasgow), crops up in the 1841 census, living in Coventry Street, Southam; by 1851 he is living in Harbury, aged sixty-three, and possibly retired.

A 'Thomas Nutt MRCS' appears with Henry Lilley Smith and Edward Welchman in the list of 'surgeons' in the town in a trade directory of 1848, and in the 1851 census he is living at 49 Oxford Street with his wife Elizabeth, whom he had married in St Mary's Church in Warwick in 1847. Elizabeth's father just happened to be John Montgomery.

The Nutt family at 49 Oxford Street in 1851 comprised Thomas (thirty-three), and Elizabeth (twenty-five), their two children, Marion (two) and Thomas (ten months), Thomas's father (seventy-one), a retired clergyman, and a nephew – a medical student – together with four servants, which included a nurse and a groom. He must have been doing pretty well in practice!

There is another shadowy medical figure in Southam: Matthew Kilpatrick, who is of more than passing interest – the earliest he appears is in 1827, when he is married in Holy Trinity Church, Long Itchington, by special licence, to Susannah Everard, spinster, of Attleborough, Nuneaton. He is described as 'Matthew Kilpatrick of Southam, surgeon' in the marriage register. Another Scot, born in Ayrshire in 1794, was he in practice in Southam? Why did he get married in Long Itchington? It wasn't Susannah's parish and they married by special licence, without calling the banns, yet he was presumably resident in Southam, and why was St James's Church considered unsuitable? Could the marriage have been urgent? Possibly, but probably not; they appear not to have had any children.

In 1835 he turns up in Rocester, a village some four miles north of Uttoxeter, apparently in practice there as a surgeon; the following advertisement appears on the front page of the *Staffordshire Advertiser* on 21st December 1839:

'Mr M F Kilpatrick, Surgeon, Oculist and Aurist, begs respectfully to intimate to the public that in future he intends to devote his attention principally to DISEASES of the EYE and EAR and may be consulted every Wednesday at Mr Everard's, Church Gate, Uttoxeter, from 11-3 o'clock. Uttoxeter, 2 Dec 1839.'

In the 1851 census (he died the following year), he describes himself as 'general practitioner, of the University of Edinborough [sic]', but a researcher of Staffordshire's medical practitioners in 1851 could not find any evidence for his Edinburgh qualification – nor indeed any qualification at all – and concluded he was 'unqualified'.

If that was indeed so, it is unthinkable that Henry Lilley Smith would have associated with him professionally – or in any way at all – whilst he was in Southam. Could that explain why he had to slink away to Long Itchington to be married?

'Oculist and Aurist' indeed – perhaps treatment of diseases of the eye and ear was an interest; indeed, he may have been influenced by Henry Lilley Smith and the work of the Southam Infirmary, or perhaps this was just an easier option for untrained full-time practice. Again, no more is known.

8

LAST YEARS

Surprisingly, Henry Lilley Smith contributed to the medical literature hardly at all, despite his disappointment that, 'Some considerable men of the best talents and observation have lived and died in great practice, without having promoted science in any great degree, or transmitted one useful fact to posterity', as he wrote in his 'Observations' pamphlet of 1819.

One would have thought his clinical enthusiasm would have led to his publishing a sheaf of case histories of interest, with suggested improvements in the treatment and management of eye diseases, as he had exhorted the profession, but he published only a single case report in the *Provincial Medical and Surgical Journal* in 1847, which is disappointing. In it he describes in physiological terms the disruption he observed – the result of an injury from a stone in infancy – to the iris and pupil of an eye of a girl, aged thirteen [see Appendix 9]. The damage was irreparable. Henry Lilley Smith regretted that the family had travelled some distance to attend the Eye Infirmary, only to be disappointed.

He was a strange man in his later years. In 1842, he had published a non-medical book with the title *A Diagram to Define the Lives of the Patriarchs, and the Early History of the Seed of the*

Serpent and the Seed of the Woman, particularly in reference to the Origin of Disease and the Danger of Unsanctified Knowledge; it was, ostensibly, a book of 'Biblical scholarship', with a number of surprising and unrelated additional chapters of self-promotion about the Coventry Self-Supporting Dispensary, the Harbury Sick Club and public holidays for the working class; but, to be honest, the first part is incomprehensible.

In 1857 he published *Lithographs representing photographs of the 'Church of the First Born' as uncovered by the 'Sun of Righteousness' to St. John, in the island of Patmos, that he might show to the 'Children of Light' things which must shortly come to pass on the opening of the Seals of the Covenant and which are necessary to be understood for their recovering the dominion over the earth, for their Lord and Master, the Second Adam.* [57]

Surely the longest book title in the world. It contained more bizarre views, which were widely ridiculed: this is the final paragraph of the review by the *Birmingham Gazette*:

'[Henry Lilley Smith] believes religious societies can do anything; he is quick at interference; he is a good hand at damning everybody; he is inclined to interfere with everything; and he devoutly believes he has got the key to every difficulty. These are high qualifications. The objection that he is manifestly deranged, we can consider to be utterly irrelevant.'

But even during this period of his life he never gave up promoting the concept of the self-supporting dispensary; in 1853 he laid out a – surprisingly, for him – succinct argument for their establishment as a distinct improvement when compared with 'the monstrous abuses of most of our medical charities' in a single-paged letter to a medical journal. It was the distillation of a lifetime's campaigning, and is quoted in full:

---

57   There is a copy in the Bodleian Library, Oxford.

OLD SYSTEM

1. Medical accounts, however moderate, are, except when sickness is of short duration, much beyond the means of the majority of working men.

2. Medical accounts not paid, or deferred till an unpleasant feeling has been created number list between patient and doctor, totally opposed to feelings of gratitude on the part of the patient, and destructive of mutual confidence, which ought to be cherished between them.

3. Quack's medicines, family physic, amateur male and female doctors or unlicensed practitioners are of necessity resorted to by the poor.

4. Improvidence, drunkenness, folly in dress, pauperism, and beggary are begotten, caressed, and encouraged by eleemosynary.[58] Dispensaries, lying-in hospitals, and all the modes of medical charity, which time-servers uphold by balls, bazaars, and all other contrivances, to gild and blazon forth the pseudo-benevolence of the frivolous and the wealthy.

5. Bottle bill, drug bill, day-book, dispenser's salary, wages to errand boy.

6. Ingratitude, faithlessness, thanklessness, degradation, idleness, and frequently loss of elective franchise.

7. Medical men are separated by jealousy, suspicion, weakness, and unfair competition; while they are likewise subjected to ceaseless toil in one dirty round of street or country duty.

NEW SYSTEM

1. Payment of one penny per week for adults, and one half-penny for children, brings the best medical advice within the reach of the poorest working men who have employment.

2. Subscriptions paid in advance; and if paid with forfeits for delay, the collector, and not the doctor, bears the obloquy.

3. Qualified practitioners of the Dispensaries are resorted to by the poor. There is no distinction of London, Dublin, Edinburgh or Glasgow, licentiates, members, or fellows. [The lives of the rich and poor are of equal value in the sight of God].

4. Provident habits, sobriety, dress suited to the station in life, and independence encouraged; and the heavenly lessons practically taught to the poor, that it is equally a duty of all to 'bear one another's burdens', and to 'provide for his own household'.

5. No surgery expenses, no bill writing, no bill delivery, no dunning, no courting.

6. Gratitude, respectability, union and thankfulness, industry, and the probability of acquiring the elective franchise.

7. Medical neighbours are brought together and made friendly, forbearing, and accommodating, by learning that they have a common interest in each other, so that they might escape occasionally from the fatigue of practice, without finding on their return that their interests had been neglected or any advantage taken of them during their absence.

---

58   A splendid word, regrettably now fallen into disuse = 'giving alms; charitable'.

There is such a great deal of sense in the above argument (ignoring the homilies), that it is difficult to understand why his model of dispensary practice was not adopted overnight by the profession. Professional paranoia, probably.

He proposed further change, adding tentatively at the foot of the letter:

'I might add to the above list many other indirect advantages likely to spring from teaching the poor to provide for sickness. One of these I will mention, namely, that provident dispensaries might be made the productive nuclei of provident banks and life assurance societies.'

Provident banks (and the like) will, regrettably, have to remain an aspect of the provident movement for discussion elsewhere…

In spite of such continued exhortations to his fellow practitioners, Henry Lilley Smith was to lose his final battle to establish another provident dispensary, this time locally, in Warwick.

It was a reasonable idea, admittedly, to mark Queen Victoria's visit to Warwick in 1858 in such a manner, and he was supported in his proposal by his son-in-law Edward Bicknell, from the Coventry Provident Dispensary, but it was pointed out by others during a meeting held in Judges' House, Warwick, on 10th July, 1858 to discuss the matter, that a Provident Sick Association was in existence in Warwick already, having been founded by the vicar of St Peter's Church the previous year, in 1857, for working men, and also 'there was already a functioning eleemosynary dispensary in the town', which had been established in 1826 (partly with the fundraising help and support of Dr John Conolly as its medical officer, then in practice in Stratford-upon-Avon).

Henry Lilley Smith's proposal for a Provident Sick Association for all was rejected. One detractor wrote in a letter published in the *Warwick Advertiser* of 12th February 1859 that he (presumably a he; the letter was signed merely '*Fiat Justitia*') suspected Henry Lilley Smith was merely 'seeking a niche in the Temple of Fame': it was further anonymous criticism, to which Henry Lilley Smith had been subjected throughout his career (and which seems to me to be just a little cowardly), and in argument merely a regurgitation of Thomas Wakley of *The Lancet*'s old criticism of doctors and their 'nepotistic puff shops' from 1829.

Be that as it may, rejection of his proposal at the meeting was a great disappointment to him, from all accounts. He was now seventy years of age, and in failing health.

Henry Lilley Smith died in his home the following year, 1859, aged seventy-one, on 11th April, and was buried in the family's tomb, after the death announcement in the *Leamington Spa Courier* of 'a funeral service in St James's Church, Southam, to be held at 5pm on Saturday 16th April'. There was no later report made by that paper, however, regarding the numbers who attended 'out of respect, affection, or merely the hope of a party'.[59] Not much likelihood of the latter, on this occasion, I fear.

For the previous two years he had suffered from 'Bright's Disease of the Kidneys', according to his death certificate.[60] During this time, as we have seen, he had still been active in medical practice: this was typical for the era – the careers of the majority of medical men were ended by death; only a fortunate few being able to retire, either on the proceeds of their practice or other good fortune (marrying into money).

But, with regards to the battle lost in 1858 for a new-style 'dispensary for all' in Warwick, he may have actually won the war, albeit posthumously: the town did later form a small-scale

---

59   Simon Loftus's observation, perhaps pertaining more to funerals in Ireland: see Bibliography.

60   'Bright's Disease' [progressive deterioration in kidney function, associated with high blood pressure] was first described in 1827 by Dr Richard Bright (1789–1858), a physician at Guy's Hospital. In the 1850s there was no effective treatment.

Provident Sick Association, which later changed its name to the Warwick Provident Society and its style of practice to that of Southam's Dispensary – although, without premises, it had to operate from the homes of the two surgeons involved. Come 1871, the charitable dispensary and the Provident Society combined, and moved into an elegant townhouse in Castle Street (which continued to house a medical practice until 2008).

In the first forty years of its existence until 1858, the year before he died, the Southam Eye and Ear Infirmary had admitted 12,200 patients, of whom two thirds were discharged 'cured', and a substantial additional number 'relieved' [see Appendix 8 for a statistical analysis, by year of admission]. For one practitioner, virtually single-handed throughout that period, it was a truly formidable achievement.

Many tributes were paid: here are three – one personal, one professional, and one from the local press.

William Fretton FSA, a Coventry historian and antiquary, wrote: 'I had the privilege of enjoying his personal acquaintance and friendship for years, and had always regarded him as a great and good man, free from many of the prejudices of his class, and ready to promote any philanthropic object.'

The Coventry Provident Dispensary noted:

'The Committee desires to record its admiration for the character, and deep respect for the memory of the late Mr Henry Lilley Smith. The Coventry Provident Dispensary, in common with all similar institutions, owes its origins to his untiring zeal and earnest heartfelt philanthropy; the Committee desires to convey to Mrs Smith and the family their sincere sorrow for a loss which will be long felt by all who are interested and occupied in promoting the well-being of the poor around them.'

The obituary published in the *Leamington Spa Courier* of 23ʳᵈ April 1859 was extensive, but, as the edited extract below indicates, a little more sanguine:

'Henry Lilley Smith's experiences as Parish Surgeon soon impressed him with a deep sense of the many claims which the poor had upon the attention and benevolence of the rich, and of the many ways in which their distresses or sufferings might be alleviated by the joint efforts of both classes. In his prospectus for the Southam Infirmary, Mr Smith stated that if he should meet with the support he anticipated, the principal energies of his professional life should be directed to the benefit of the poor who might be recommended to his care. The whole of his subsequent life was an admirable and continuous fulfilment of this pledge.

We can remember the time when he was not favourably received by his fellow brethren. His Infirmary was a special hospital and his skill was derived from it; and the renown of his cures brought patients from every part of the midlands to the little town of Southam.

But to the majority he was an alarmist; his intense earnestness, suave deportment, with a slight eccentricity of manner and trifling defects of language, stamped his personality more strongly on the memory. His celebrity continued to increase, and his Infirmary was successful.

This led, as the knowledge of the institution extended, to his being consulted by a wealthier class, which caused an outcry by other medical men that his practice was interfering in an improper manner and to their detriment. Despite such accusations being overborne by the honourable and philanthropic conduct of Mr Smith, they were from time to time revived throughout his life, and tinged with bitterness and grief some of the last hours of Mr Smith's life.

It was not only as a medical man, but as a philanthropist, that Mr Smith was known to the public. The worthy began to perceive his worth, and the charitable to desire to be associated with him.'

Perhaps he was a more kindly and tolerant man in day-to-day conversation than the legacy of much of his written works (and the only surviving photograph) might suggest.

A memorial to him was established in the form of an Endowment Fund, which by 12th September 1859, when the list of donors was published, had received £3,654 8s. 0d. *in toto* from ninety-six subscribers, of whom thirty-one were members of the clergy (but whose contributions amounted to a mere 3% of the total sum collected).

9

HENRY LILLEY SMITH'S LEGACY

After Henry Lilley Smith's death, his private residence, stables and gardens were sold by his son, the Revd William Lilley Smith, to the Committee administering the Institution on 25th May 1860 for £1,250; a Memorial Trust was formed, and a memorial plaque with the following inscription was prominently placed on the front of the Infirmary, still clearly evident in the photograph of the building as it is today:

Eye and Ear Infirmary

These premises were purchased AD MDCCCLX
as a MEMORIAL to
Henry Lilley Smith M.R.C.S.
and are held in trust for the purposes of this Infirmary
founded by him AD MDCCCVIII
and fostered by his attendance and skill
for upward of forty years

His widow, and daughter Sophia, moved into a house belonging to William, which stood in the paddock behind 'Walton's Close', but which is now demolished.

According to an undated handwritten article in the possession of Southam Heritage, 'they lived there and had a French maid who committed suicide, and, not being permitted to be buried in consecrated ground, was buried in the paddock near the river. Part of a gravestone erected to her memory (it is said by the Sisters of the Convent) was dug up during work near the river bank.'[61]

*

The Dispensary ceased to function – no successor being found who was willing to take over the duties of dispenser (and I sense the other medical men of the town weren't particularly anxious to become involved with it either) – and the cottage slowly became derelict, eventually to be demolished in 1868.

However, the Infirmary survived, albeit with a new role in the life of the town. In spite of Southam being situated at the junction of five turnpike roads, which had brought a degree of prosperity to the town in the early 1800s, after 1851 it became increasingly isolated when the London North Western Railway's new railway line from Rugby to Leamington and GWR's railway line to Leamington came into being. The railways provided passengers with rapid, convenient travel, protected from the elements and three times faster (and far more comfortable) than the same journey by coach, but in so doing, both new railway lines bypassed Southam, the nearest stations being either Depper's

---

61   Our Lady's Convent, on the corner of Wood Street and Daventry Street, was established in 1876 by the 'Sisters of the Poor Child Jesus'. Originally a Catholic order from Aachen, Germany, the nuns were dedicated to the education of poor, orphan, and destitute children. In 1902, they built behind the Convent an imposing orphanage-cum-boarding school for girls; one of the most imposing buildings in the town, it was demolished in 1991, to be replaced by 'The Cloisters', a development of private houses. The Convent today is a retreat house and the order is very much depleted in numbers.

Bridge or Marton – both some miles from the town. Despite the railway companies providing 'horsed buses' up to four times a day between these stations and Southam, the towns of Rugby and Northampton were no longer convenient catchment areas for Eye Infirmary patients – indeed, Henry Lilley Smith had remarked on this reduction in patients from the Northampton area in an annual report, just a few years before he died – but, on the other hand, an increased need for the provision of general medical care for the local populace arose. The Committee therefore decided to add the facilities of a cottage hospital to the Eye and Ear Infirmary.

Two surgeons were appointed to the newly styled 'Southam Infirmary and Cottage Hospital'. One was Edward Ruttledge, from the Wood Street practice in the town, the other was a new arrival in Southam, Mr David Rice. Trained in Leeds and qualified MRCS in 1861, he joined the Infirmary in 1862 and later moved into Mrs Smith's house after she and Sophia had joined William in Dorsington Rectory.

The existing number of beds in the Infirmary were considered to be 'insufficient for the wants of the place', so in 1863, Henry Lilley Smith's house adjoining the Infirmary was altered and enlarged at a cost of £400, 'to provide large airy day rooms and splendid wards, for the removal of all cases of sickness from the crowded cottages of the poor, to afford succour in cases of accident, and provide accommodation in case the ordinary patients of the Infirmary fall ill.' (*Leamington Spa Courier*, 20th November 1869.)

But William Lilley Smith, who appears to have inherited something of his father's temperament, was unhappy with this course of events:

'My father's services [to the Infirmary] had been entirely gratuitous,' he wrote in the *Leamington Spa Courier* of 4th December 1869, 'but as it was felt this could not be expected of a future medical officer, it was intended that his house should provide rented accommodation (and a source of income to the Infirmary) for the medical officer. The house was then converted to sick wards for general cases. The alterations have been very painful to the feelings of my father's family.'

The disquiet between the Committee and the Lilley Smith family about the new cottage hospital development of the Infirmary became personal – always a sign of desperation – which circulated via the correspondence columns of the *Leamington Spa Courier*; never the best medium to reach a *rapprochement* in an adult manner. David Rice was caught in the crossfire, being criticised in print for having 'no special ophthalmological surgical skills', but his defendants countered such criticism by informing them that 'he was a pupil of Mr Nunnerly [sic], the eminent oculist of Leeds, and the late Sir William Lawrence, the most celebrated surgeon in London of his day, has borne testimony to the skill of Mr Rice as an operator.'[62]

This display of parish pump politics exasperated Edward Ruttledge to the extent that the *Courier* reported he 'somewhat hastily, threw up his appointment' and Henry Blenkinsop MRCS, the surgeon to Warwick Dispensary and Union, was appointed 'Honorary Surgeon' to the Infirmary in his stead.[63]

Mr Rice however remained in post at the Infirmary in Southam during this period; I presume he merely maintained a dignified silence during this *contretemps,* for by 1875, he had

---

62   Thomas Nunneley (1809–1870), MRCS, eye surgeon, Eye and Ear Infirmary, Leeds, which functioned from 1822–1869 (an almost identical lifespan to Southam's).
Sir William Lawrence (1783–1867), FRCS, eye surgeon, Bart's and Bedlam Hospitals, and later President of the Royal College of Surgeons.

63   Henry Blenkinsop (1813–1866), FRCS; trained at St Bartholomew's Hospital; surgeon to Warwick Dispensary and the County Gaol, and Medical Officer to Warwick Union workhouse. His prominent chest-tomb is in the churchyard on the N. side of St Mary's Church, Warwick, close to the footpath that leads to The Butts.

moved into 'The Abbey' (originally a Jacobean mansion and now Grade ll listed, it remains the most imposing house in Southam), so his work must have been respected and by then he was clearly well established in the town.

Plainly, it was not a happy time, but tempers settled and after Henry Blenkinsop died in 1866, Edward Ruttledge must have been forgiven his hasty resignation and reappointed, for according to the medical directories of the time, he was living from 1863 until 1865 in Faringdon, Berkshire (where he had been born), and returned to Southam to 'Warwick Road' in 1866, where he remained until 1875.[64]

The Committee of the newly refurbished and extended Infirmary advertised (ever the optimist) for patients in the *Northampton Mercury* in December 1870, adding 'Domestic management is entrusted to a lady well qualified for the duties of her post by a course of training in a large City Hospital.'

The final sentence of the advertisement stated, 'Subscriptions are urgently needed to enable the Committee to extend the benefits which the Institution is capable of affording', which was a touch ominous.

And so it proved. The Infirmary's new life was indeed short-lived; it closed to patients in 1872, a mere two years later, due to lack of funds, despite repeated attempts at fundraising.

William Lilley Smith later wrote on the back of a report of the accounts of the Infirmary for 1870, now in the Record Office, which documents donations totalling £991.12s. 0d towards a building fund:

'Very many of the largest donors on the list were old friends and supporters of my father's Eye and Ear Infirmary and we felt grieved that the amount contributed was being expended

---

64   In the Medical Register of 1876, his address was 28 Finsbury Square, London: on leaving Southam, he appears to have joined the army; he died in 1878, aged forty-four, at Salonika, from typhoid.

so lavishly and unwisely on building alterations.[65] [And yet the building's frontage today looks very like it was in Henry Lilley Smith's lifetime, if compared with the engraving made when the dispensary was still in good repair.]

This relates to the effort made to change the Infirmary into a general Cottage Hospital and it was done with such a large and ill-advised expenditure in alterations and new building which latter was calculated to depreciate the value of the house adjoining which at that time still belonged to me that I remonstrated and as the plan for the new building was persisted in I had the damages to me surveyed by Mr Allen, architect of Stratford, and sent in a claim for compensation to the Committee.

The reasonableness of this was acknowledged but there remained no funds in their hands and eventually I found it desirable to sell my remaining property to their nominee, Mr Rice, then surgeon to the Institution.

However, the overlay had been so great of capital, and the promised annual subscriptions being inadequate, the institution collapsed and upon application being made to the Charity Commissioners in 1878 a scheme was authorised by them and trustees appointed for the further management of the Charity.'

Southam's expanded cottage hospital had existed for merely ten years, before its closure in 1872: the nearest hospitals were then all some distance away – at Leamington, Warwick, or Northampton – so continued access to beds would have been very useful indeed for the town's practitioners.

A journey to hospital in those days can't have been much fun: on 25th September 1854, a farm labourer was brought to the

---

65   Donors included four surgeons, twenty-four members of the clergy and of the great and the good, seven knights of the realm, two lords and two earls. No physicians donated.

County Asylum at Hatton for admission (with the relevant Order for Admission correctly completed), 'strongly strapped down in the bottom of a cart'. I suspect this mode of transport of the sick (in body or in mind) was not unusual; it may well be that – given the choice between home or hospital – many of Southam's patients would have preferred to have taken their chances and remained at home.

Other nearby towns also came to realise beds locally were an asset, and cottage hospitals would be established at Brackley (1876), Shipston-on-Stour (1896) and Chipping Norton (1914). All are still functioning today within the NHS (if somewhat precariously, and at Brackley admittedly in name only), albeit with fewer in-patient beds but much expanded diagnostic and day-care services as 'Community Hospitals'.[66]

As William Lilley Smith stated, following the hospital's closure, the 'Southam Eye and Ear Infirmary and Cottage Hospital Charity' was formed, trustees were appointed to run it, and in 1880 the building – by then known as 'The Laurels' – was being let to the 'Southam Institute and Club' as a meeting place-cum-parish hall.

*

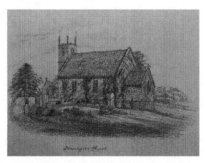

Illustration 14: St. Peter's Church, Dorsington 1871 – drawing by Sophia Smith

---

66   Brackley Cottage Hospital closed in 1996, to become a private nursing home. A 'Community Hospital' opened in 2021, part of the new premises of the town's medical practice.

Henry Lilley Smith's widow Mary and her daughter Sophia had moved from the small cottage (long gone) near the site of the dispensary by 1871, to live with William near Stratford-upon-Avon: he had been appointed Rector of St Peter's Church, Dorsington, in 1866.

For all three, this proved to be their final home: Mary died in the Rectory on 19th January 1877, aged eighty-four, following 'Bronchitis three days' according to the death certificate, and was buried in the family's tomb in Southam on 26th January 1877. William and Sophia lived on with a cook and a servant, until Sophia died, aged fifty-three, on 21st December 1888. The cause of death was recorded as:

'Valvular disease of heart (years)
Dropsy (2 months)
Syncope
(signed) C E Hobbes LRCP' [67]

She too was buried in the family tomb on 28th December 1888. Her relatively early age of death suggests she probably had rheumatic heart disease and was increasingly invalid therefrom, dying from progressive cardiac failure or 'dropsy'.

Her will of 27th April 1877 (witnessed by Stewart Lynch, the curate at Dorsington, and Emma Sanders, Dorsington's schoolmistress) contained one clause of some interest to us: she requested – if her brother William Lilley Smith were to die before her – 'that £4,000 be employed by the trustees of the Smith Memorial Charity to establish in the Smith Memorial Buildings at Southam an Industrial Provident Home for the Blind in memory of Henry Lilley Smith as the Charity Commissioners shall authorize, but if said trustees shall not be able to obtain the authority then the £4,000 to be part of the general property and income applied as authorized by the Charity Commissioners.'

---

67   Charles Edward Hobbes MRCS, LRCP(Ed), LSA, (1874), a local practitioner from Bidford, near Stratford-upon-Avon.

However, William outlived her and thus the bequest became void.

At the time of the 1891 census, some three years later, William was still living in the Rectory, and presumably continuing to diligently discharge his duties as Rector. He lived there with two servants and two lodgers; one, Stuart Lynch, then aged sixty-one, was the curate at Dorsington from 1884 until 1892, and the other was a nephew, George Bicknell, in his twenties, then describing himself as a 'farming pupil', presumably under instruction at Moat House Farm, Dorsington, which was owned by William Lilley Smith.[68]

It must have come as a very great surprise to everyone to read in the *Leamington Spa Courier* of 23rd March 1895 the following report:

'DORSINGTON Death of the Rector – On Wednesday last [the Revd William Lilley Smith] was discovered missing from his home in Dorsington, and a note was found, in which he stated that he contemplated suicide by drowning himself in the river Avon. Dragging operations were commenced and the body found.

For twenty years or more he was Guardian for Dorsington on the Stratford-upon-Avon Board of Governors [of the Stratford Union workhouse]. He was a man of considerable intellectual achievements and he was a Scholar of Trinity College, Cambridge. It is believed by his friends that his mind had become unhinged by close study, and it is stated that about twelve years ago some anxiety was felt for his safety because of his erratic conduct. Mr Smith was of a very kindly disposition and sympathetic nature.'

---

68   George Bicknell's father, Charles, was a brother of Mary (wife to Henry Lilley Smith) and a farmer and auctioneer in Caernarvonshire: George inherited Moat House Farm from William Lilley Smith after his death in 1895; by 1897 he was describing himself as a 'gentleman of private means'. The wheel of fortune.

'Unhinged by close study' may refer to his authorship of a book which had been published the previous year, entitled *Historical Notices and Recollections relating to the Parish of Southam, In the County of Warwick, together with the Parochial Registers from AD 1539 and Churchwardens' Accounts AD 1580*; it was illustrated with pen and ink drawings 'of its most interesting objects and scenery', by his sister Sophia.

It was the work of a typical Victorian 'gentleman scholar'; for the main part it contained his copies of transcripts made by Southam's then parish clerk, William Basse, in the 1790s, from the original parish records held in the church. They included the register of baptisms from January 1539–May 1601, the register of marriages from April 1539–November 1630, and the churchwarden's accounts from 1580–1603, together with commentaries of his own, which were mainly explanations of ecclesiastical terms and events in the ecclesiastical calendar. To these he added observations on the history of the parish, and a contributor, Willoughby Gardner FLS, FRGS, a noted antiquarian and archaeologist of the time (and distant family relative), wrote additional chapters on genealogy, geology and various aspects of the natural history of the locality.

The coroner's inquest revealed that 'the Reverend Lilley Smith had slept in his bed the previous night, and had gone out on the morning of his death fully dressed. On the bedside table was a small piece of paper, found under the deceased's watch and written upon it in pencil in the Reverend gentleman's handwriting were the words "in the river at Welford Pastures". There the body was recovered from the river fully dressed, boots laced, no marks of violence.'

The verdict was 'Suicide, whilst temporarily insane'.

The funeral procession, on 26th March 1895, commenced in Dorsington Church, and processed to Southam; then followed a burial service in St James's Church, Southam, with interment in the family tomb.

It is noteworthy that the Revd Lilley Smith was allowed to be laid to rest in consecrated ground, but his mother's anonymous

French maid (no more is known about her) was not; it may well have been that her religious persuasion was Roman Catholic, and canon law was applied to her for her transgressions (this would eventually be relaxed in the 1980s). The Church of England, however, had taken a more sympathetic view regarding those who had taken their own life about a hundred years earlier, and permitted burial in consecrated ground.

Be that as it may, there still remains the uncomfortable sense of there being 'one law for the rich; another law for the poor'.

*

The Infirmary Charity's Minute Book from 1877–1965 has survived, documenting its decisions and events from 1877, including its amalgamation with Southam United Charities in 1953, up to its eventual closure.

It appears to have been run conscientiously throughout these years, with only four or five long-serving chairmen for the almost 100 years of its existence, with no evidence of any of the internal disquiet of the 1860s. It tried to carry on Henry Lilley Smith's practice and ideals as far as possible, and the Charity Commissioners' directive, by continuing to make substantial annual subscriptions to the Warneford Hospital in Leamington and the Birmingham Eye Hospital.

In 1889, William Lilley Smith had approached the Trustees, offering the Trust an oil painting of his father, and with a request to place a memorial near the site of the original Dispensary, at his own expense. Both offers were accepted; the oil painting was lent to the tenant of the Infirmary for safe keeping (and display therein) and the memorial was duly constructed, and unveiled on 29th September 1889.

*

Now the traveller comes to the fourth side of the monument, with its inscription:

IN THE YEAR 1895
A BEQUEST OF £3000 WAS
LEFT TO THE TRUSTEES OF
THE SMITH MEMORIAL CHARITY
SOUTHAM
BY THE TWO CHILDREN OF THE
FOUNDER IN PIOUS MEMORY
OF THEIR FATHER & MOTHER
AND IN ORDER TO ENABLE
THE TRUSTEES TO REOPEN
THE INSTITUTION FOR THE
BENEFIT OF THIS TOWN
AND NEIGHBOURHOOD

In William Lilley Smith's will dated 2nd March 1893, some two years – almost to the day – before he immersed himself in the River Avon, he bequeathed 'to the Trustees of the Smith Memorial Charity £3000 towards establishing in the buildings a sanatorium and nursing home in connection with the Warneford Hospital if possible, if not, some other hospital or, if not, to general interests of the Institution; upon condition that they place on the stone pedestal, erected by the testator in the grounds of the Institution to mark the site of the first Provident Dispensary in the United Kingdom, the inscription [as above] he has directed to be so placed', and he also gave the Trust 'a further £200, the income therefrom to be applied on keeping in good repair the memorial stone upon the Infirmary buildings and the pedestal lately erected by himself.'

The income from the bequest 'was also to provide a yearly sum of no less than £25 and no more than £35 towards the maintenance of a nurse for the benefit of the poor of the parish and neighbourhood'.

He had been adamant that the financial collapse of the Infirmary after his father's death had been due to its overexpansion to include a Cottage Hospital, and was probably hoping that combining its activities with established hospitals in the area would resurrect it. But it was not to be: the wished-for resurrection of the buildings into 'a sanatorium and nursing home', and commemorated as such on the memorial stone, never materialised. But the Infirmary did not reopen: the Charity Commissioners considered it was not practicable, so, in 1898, it was decided that the building should continue to be let, and any income the Trust accrued from the letting, together with the interest of the £3,000 'William Lilley Smith Charity (general)' be used to support 'any Hospital or Infirmary in England and Wales established for the treatment of diseases of the Eye and Ear, or for benefit of any General Hospital or Infirmary in England and Wales for deserving poor persons' and the £200 'William Lilley Smith Charity (memorial)' bequest should be used, as intended, for upkeep of the memorial.

In addition to subscriptions to the Warneford Hospital and the Birmingham Eye Hospital, the Trust also subscribed to the Birmingham Ear, Nose & Throat Hospital (1891) and the Birmingham Skin Hospital (1881), and – sporadically – the Droitwich Brine Baths (a spa since 1836), presumably when there were patients in the town requiring that specific treatment.[69]

The part nurses had to play in the activities of the Infirmary and Dispensary has not yet been addressed, and indeed the history of the district nurse in Southam has also yet to be written (once again, regrettably, this isn't it), but they formed an integral part of the success of both establishments. In the

---

69   The Birmingham Skin Hospital, in John Bright Street, opened originally in 1881 as the 'Skin & Lock Hospital' (Lock Hospitals were specifically for venereal diseases). It was later more discreetly known as the 'Skin and Urinary Diseases Hospital'. Its earlier functions were still plainly evident to those in the know: the entrance for women and children patients was at the front of the building, the entrance for men was at the rear.

1831 abstract of his plan for Self-Supporting Charitable and Parochial Dispensaries, presented at Sackville Street, London, Henry Lilley Smith advised:

> 'In long illnesses [Free Members] may perhaps be supplied with a nurse, cordials, food, linen etc., ... the extra supplies to patients in sickness to be allowed under the direction of a Visiting Committee, and chiefly, if not entirely, to Members of the Free Class.'

The Southam Dispensary reports made mention of a 'Visiting Committee', which may well have included ladies, but not a 'Ladies Committee' *per se*; Atherstone Dispensary, however, raised a fund from donations and subscriptions of Honorary Members, 'to assist the deserving and industrious Free Members in sickness. The fund was employed in supplying Cordials and Linen *gratis*, and paying nurses appointed under the direction of the Medical Men, assisted by a Committee of Ladies.'

After one year of activity, Atherstone reported in 1829 that:

> 'The Ladies Committee have acted with a discretion and zeal that has attracted general admiration. They have visited regularly and impartially the Free Members, and have gained a salutary influence over them, which, without the regulations and system of this dispensary they could not have obtained. The discreet use of this power constitutes one of the leading traits of this Charity; for it is by this means made evident to the honest and industrious that the desire of their superiors is to raise them, and to promote the happiness of them and their children.'

Nursing is an ancient profession, of course, then mainly carried out in a hospital or other institutional environment. One hundred years earlier or thereabouts, the Governors of Westminster

Hospital (England's first charitable hospital), in 1742, had found its nurses to be a boisterous bunch, noting that occasionally they had to be reprimanded or even dismissed 'for drinking or staying out all night or tempting the porter or the apothecary's pupil.' (Lucky apothecary's pupil.)

There had been a discussion in an editorial of the *London Medical Repository and Review* of March 1826 regarding forming an English Protestant version of the French Catholic order of the 'Sisters of Charity', who acted in France very much in the capacity of district nurses, aided by financial support from the French government.

'These good women are seen at all hours of the day going about in quest of proper objects of their pious duties,' it wrote. 'They are persons of respectable station, sometimes even of a certain *rank* [their italics] and have always acquired sufficient information to make them useful without being officious.' But, regrettably, nothing came of it.

'Ladies' had inspected monthly the housekeeping accounts of the Infirmary since its inception: nurses accompanied Henry Lilley Smith and John Gardner when they attended the cholera victims in Southam in the 1832 epidemic, but they were more likely to have come from the 'Ladies Bountiful' (his term) end of the spectrum, such as monitored the housekeeping of the Infirmary, rather than the 'Westminster Hospital end' (mine), so to speak.

At this distance in time it is impossible to discover what Southam's Dispensary nurses actually did, but it is likely that their function was limited to 'supplying cordials and linen *gratis*', as reported, but may possibly have included changing surgical dressings and applying leeches etc., although that might well have been considered indecorous behaviour for a young, unmarried woman in the 1830s; it was more likely that storage and transportation of leeches and their application would have been the province of the apothecary or doctor and changing dressings, washing and feeding a patient was more usually the responsibility of a (female) member of the family.

The Commissioners in Lunacy reported in 1856 that in the nation's workhouses, 'the attendants for the most part are Pauper Inmates totally unfit for the charge imposed upon them. The wards are gloomy, and unprovided with any means for occupation, exercise or amusement.'

By 1890 there was one paid nurse in the Southam workhouse, supervising a sick ward of eighteen beds, but that was long after Henry Lilley Smith's time, and even so, her duties would still have been, for the most part, feeding the sick, tidying the ward, mending bed linen and uniforms. It is highly unlikely anyone would try and engineer their admission to the workhouse purely for access to nursing care: whilst the nurse may have been paid, she would probably have been only rudimentarily trained, if at all.

District nursing 'for the benefit of the poor in the parish and neighbourhood', using the Revd William Lilley Smith's phrase, became quite well established locally in the years following his father's demise.

Locally, the Stratford-upon-Avon Nursing Institute had been founded in 1872 by their Lady Superintendent for twenty years, Emily Minet, which became the Stratford-upon-Avon Nursing Home for Convalescent Women and Sick Children in 1873; it only ministered to patients in their homes within the town, and managed to live harmoniously with the Stratford Infirmary (which admitted neither of the Nursing Home's two groups of patients). The nurses were recruited mainly from domestic servants, who were 'used to taking orders, were deferential and accustomed to hard work', and hospital trained in Birmingham for a year. Was this the right approach? The *British Medical Journal* thought so in 1890:

'Ladies [of the upper and middle classes], as a rule, do not make first-rate nurses... ladies take to nursing from slightly morbid reasons; they are 'disappointed', or they want something with which to kill the *ennui*, or they have religious convictions on the subject.'

There were about seven trained and two 'probationer nurses' at any one time; their competence was highly regarded and they ministered to the sick poor within the town *gratis*, income for this coming from the fees charged to inpatients of the nursing home and from private patients; it was not unusual for a nurse to be sent many miles away to live in 'as a trusted servant' with a family for the duration of an episode of illness. There is a memorial to Emily Minet – a stained-glass window – in Holy Trinity Church, Stratford-upon-Avon.

Nursing funds developed locally in the more rural areas to provide some district nursing care on a modest scale, and the 'Southam and District Nursing Fund' must have been one of the earlier ones established, for there is a grave in the churchyard of St James's Church (now unidentifiable), but which was originally marked with a headstone inscribed:

'Sarah Carter Hodges
Died 30th September 1901 aged 67
This stone erected
in appreciation of her kindness
by many friends at Southam'

Born in Avon Dassett in 1835, after marriage she had lived in Banbury Road with her husband Samuel, a 'cement worker', and their five children, and been a nurse for many years to the town's populace.

But following Sarah Carter Hodges' death, the 'Southam and District Nursing Fund' appears to have fallen upon hard times, for that same year it asked the Trustees of the 'Southam Infirmary and Cottage Hospital Charity' for financial assistance – 'if their Committee's funds and services were put at the Trustees' disposal'.

The Trustees decided to allow their continued autonomy, merely inviting a sub-committee of three members from the Southam Nursing Fund Committee to join their annual meetings, and supported them by making annual donations to the Nursing

Fund in accordance with William Lilley Smith's bequest; in fact the Trust became its largest subscriber. Other local 'Nursing Funds' also received (more modest) annual donations: the 'Lady Knightley Byfield Nursing Club' from 1901,[70] 'Harbury and District Nurses Fund' from 1903, and 'Stockton District Nurses Fund' from 1908 – they would all become 'Nursing Associations' after 1916, run on provident lines, together with 'Napton & Shuckborough Nursing Association' from 1922 and 'Long Itchington Nursing Association' from 1932. Annual subscriptions continued until the establishment of the NHS.

Accounts for the 'Southam Nursing Association' survive for 1926 and 1927: by then running on provident lines, it had 153 members, each paying 8s. 8d. annually, which allowed 'services of the Nurse for all ordinary cases of illness, except those requiring isolation'. This covered the subscriber's husband or wife and dependants under the age of sixteen. Other members of a household could join for 1d. per week. An additional 21s. [1 gn] paid for 'the Nurse's attendance at confinement (with a doctor) and ten days post-natal nursing. Non-Subscribers will pay Double Fees'. The report goes on:

'The committee received, with much regret, Nurse Hay's resignation, for during the seventeen months she has been in Southam, her excellent work and quiet tact had won universal regard. In the meanwhile, Nurse Lovell was appointed District Nurse for three months, and in December the appointment was made permanent. The Committee felt it fortunate that the services of one so well-known and so much liked were to be obtained.'[71]

---

70   Lady Knightley of Fawsley Hall also established Badby School in 1812 'for the education of twelve poor girls'.

71   Many charitable nursing institutions became provident associations in the early 1900s, influenced by Dr Jamieson Hurry's book *District Nursing on a Provident Basis*, published in 1898.

Mrs Ellen Lovell had been a resident of the town for some years before her appointment.

By the 1920s almost all rural areas in England had a local 'nurse-midwife' – in essence a qualified midwife with additional basic home nursing training; after 1948, the roles of nurse and midwife would become separated in the NHS. This diluted the number of available trained nurses at a stroke, and it took many years for trained nurse numbers to recover: in 1955, out of 9,000 district nurses employed in the NHS, about half had been trained by regional centres of the Queen's Nursing Institute (founded by Queen Victoria in 1889) but the other half had no recognised qualification at all.

*

By 1907, income from the charities' capital was very limited, and Margetts & Co, Estate agents in Warwick were asked to put the building up for sale by auction, with a clause in the deeds of sale reserving 'a 15-foot square area of land at the SW corner of the grounds of the Infirmary building facing the road' for a new site for the memorial of 1889 – which is where it now stands. The sale of the building achieved £610 0s. 0d, which was invested in the name of the Official Trustees of Charitable Funds, and it became a private dwelling. The painting of Henry Lilley Smith within it was returned to the Clerk of the Trustees (but its present whereabouts are unknown).

The Trustees now had little to do, but they continued to fund £4. 0s. 0d. *per annum* to a succession of caretakers for the upkeep of the memorial, and also continued all the annual subscriptions, until that was no longer necessary with the introduction of the NHS in 1948.

With the introduction of the National Insurance Act in 1911, the Trustees approached the Charity Commissioners suggesting their income might be used 'in cash or in kind for persons in receipt of National Assistance', but the Commissioners thought otherwise and advised the income should continue to be distributed as heretofore. Then in 1952, the Charity Commissioners suggested that in future, income of the charity should be paid quarterly to the Trustees of the 'Southam United Charity', apart from the 'memorial upkeep' fund. Occasionally, somehow, grants were still given, mainly to the Southam Infant Welfare Centre (whose premises were a temporary hut in Craven Lane well into the 1970s) for repairs or items of medical equipment, and once, in 1960, for 'adding two dials at £130 & £145 to the church clock'.

By 1965, apart from annual payments of £4 0s. 0d. for the maintenance of the memorial, the sole entry in the Minutes Book at the Trustees Annual General Meeting for the previous four years had been 'no business', and there are no further entries after 1965.

*

The lifetimes of the Infirmary and Dispensary in Southam were now over, but provident dispensaries had continued to appear throughout the country. The first of such in London had opened in St Marylebone in 1833; others followed quickly, notably, in 1854, the Clapham General and Provident Dispensary opened in a very fine 'Italianate' building, built at the height of the provident dispensary movement, and designed by its architect *gratis*.[72]

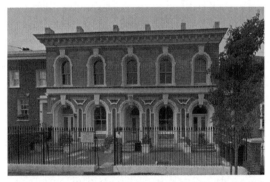

Illustration 15: Clapham Dispensary, built in 1854, at the height of the Provident Dispensary movement.

---

72   Now a Grade II listed building, it has been occupied by the London Russian Ballet School since 2005.

By 1870, some twenty dispensaries were in existence. In that year, Mr P H Holland, a Manchester surgeon, wrote in 'An Essay on Dispensaries' that he was almost drummed out of the local Medical Society in 1838 for advocating provident dispensaries: '... they were said to be "derogatory" and "bad in principle" – a general term which people used when they did not know what were their grounds for objecting.'

But by now it was widely considered that the provident dispensary system was fair and just: John Anderson MD, Medical Officer to the Haverstock Hill Dispensary in Hampstead in his lecture of 1870 'On Provident Dispensaries; their object and practical working', even went so far as to say that 'Provident Dispensary patients are less exacting and more grateful and more thoughtful of their doctor than charitable dispensary patients, and I could quote the opinion of many [other doctors] to the same effect.'

The movement was gaining momentum: even the Medical Gazette waxed lyrical: '... the direct benefits arising [from a provident dispensary], to those who have embraced it, are no more auspicious than the benefit it confers upon the profession, and the invaluable boon it bestows on the country at large, in the shape of sober, steady and provident citizens.'

By the 1880s, a provident dispensary for the medical care of the working class was considered 'best practice', and the Metropolitan Provident Medical Association was founded in 1881 to provide 'medical treatment for lower-middle-class working people'. Its intention was to provide fifty dispensaries throughout the metropolis. As ever, there was reluctance to take part by some doctors, who felt they were being 'short-changed' by the system, and although by the end of the century in London there were forty-six dispensaries in toto, Lloyd George's National Insurance Act of 1911 would replace much of the provident dispensaries' work.

His Act proposed that all workers over the age of sixteen and earning less than £160 per annum would pay 4d. (3d. if female) per week into the scheme. Employers would add 3d. and the Government would add 2d. from general taxation and the scheme would be administered by a number of 'Approved Societies'.

The scheme would provide free medical attention, including the cost of medicine, for all those contributing. Treatment would be provided by a 'panel doctor'. Contributors were also guaranteed 10s. a week for thirteen weeks of sickness and 5s. a week for a further thirteen weeks.

It was to be compulsory, each member of the workforce contributing individually to this 'ninepence for fourpence' scheme: it was the Treasury's view that 'working people ought to pay something. It gives them a feeling of self-respect and what costs nothing is not valued'. Henry Lilley Smith's sentiments entirely.

In introducing the Bill in the House of Commons on 4th May 1911, Lloyd George said:

'When a workman falls ill, if he has no provision made for him, he hangs on as long as he can and until he gets very much worse. Then he goes to a doctor and runs up a bill, and when he gets well he does his very best to pay that and the other bills. He very often fails to do so. I have met many doctors who have told me that they have hundreds of pounds of bad debts of this kind which they could not think of pressing for payment of.'

Compare this with the Second Annual Report of the Southam Dispensary published on 25th October 1825:

'It appears the subscribers are persons whose earnings are adequate to their ordinary support, but are too limited to defray the expenses of medical attendance in case of sickness in their own homes. These persons, had they been visited by sickness, must consequently have been driven to one or other of these inconveniences

– either they must have had recourse to their parishes for assistance – or they must have incurred bills, which according to the customary practice would not have been improperly charged, but which the patients had not the means to pay – or they must have foregone medical aid completely in many cases where it might have been available:– from every one of these inconveniences, it is obviously desirable, on the score of true benevolence, to rescue the labouring classes.'

Provident dispensaries declined in importance with the introduction of the 'panel doctor', but some continued, providing treatment to women, children and the elderly who were not insured under the 1911 Act; then came the abolition of the New Poor Law with the 1834 Poor Law (Amendment) Act in 1929, bringing with it the demise of the workhouse. Responsibility for care of the poor and elderly passed to county councils, and workhouses became Public Assistance Institutions, run under less severe conditions than before.

The 1948 National Assistance Act led to most workhouses being either demolished or adopted by Social Services, as homes for the elderly or hostels; some workhouses and the few remaining workhouse infirmaries were absorbed into the NHS as hospitals, although the stigma of their previous function would remain in the eye of the populace for many years.

Although the provident dispensaries were eventually superseded by the 'panel doctor', I expect that, had he still been alive, Henry Lilley Smith would have been very gratified that his proposals for affordable health care for the labouring classes and their families had eventually been adopted as national policy; but no doubt he would also have wagged his finger under your nose, emphasising that nearly a century had passed since he had opened his provident dispensary on Warwick Road – 'the first in the Kingdom'.

Appendix 1

CURRENCY CONVERSION CHART

British currency was in pounds (£), each comprised of 20 shillings (s.), each of which comprised of 12 pence (d.) until conversion to decimal coinage in 1971.

The following conversion chart may be helpful:

£	s.	d.	£	p
0	0	1	0	0.42 (approx.)
0	0	3	0	1.26 (approx.)
0	0	6	0	2.5 (approx.)
0	1	0	0	5
0	2	0	0	10
0	5	0	0	25
0	10	0	0	50

A 'guinea', or 1 gn (£1 1s. 0d.), was equivalent to £1.05; commonly used by the professions as a unit of currency.

£1 in 1810 would be worth about £50 today.

Appendix 2

(a) Itemised account for Poor attended by Mr Henry Lilley Smith according to the Orders of Mr Pridmore, Guardian of the Poor for the Parish of Southam (December 30th 1814–29th March 1815).

The Parish of Southam
1814

Dec			£. s. d.
30	two large boxes of Ointment for the Itch	Young Canning	2. 0
	three Purging Powders		1. 6
Jan			
1	an Opening Bolus & Emetic Powder	Mrs Williams	1. 6
6	an Emetic Powder -/6 & 1 Bolus 1/-		1. 6
9	twelve Powders 3/- a Mixture 2/- Emetic	Master Smith	5. 6
12	two boxes of Itch Ointment	Young Canning	2. 0
	eight Powders pint Mixture		7. 6
14	Bleeding 1/- pint Mixture box of Pills		6. 6
	Anodyne Powder	Master Rainbow	0. 6
	a Mixture and Blister		3. 6
15	box of Ointment and Powder		1. 6
16	pint Mixture	Master Smith	4. 0
	Opening an abcess on the foot	Walker's Daughter	0. 0
	Dressing – Ointments – Plasters etc		5. 0
	three Purging Powders		1. 6
17	Purging Powder	Mrs Rodknight	0. 6

18	Purging Powder	Master Smith	0. 6
	three Powders – pint Mixture, box of Pills		
		Mrs Rodknight	6. 6
19	a dose of Opening Pills	Mary Purser	0. 6
	three Leeches (use of)		2. 6
	a Night Powder		0. 6
	Opening Pills	Mrs Rodknight	0. 6
	Purging Powder	Master Walker	0. 6
	four Pills		0. 6
21	pint Mixture – three Powders –	Master Smith	0. 6
	dose of Pills	Mrs Rainbow	0. 6
	dose of Pills	Mary Semple	0. 6
	paper of Pills	Old Phillips	1. 0
	pint Mixture & Powder	Mrs Rodknight	4. 6
22	a Mixture	Mary Semple	2. 0
		Carried forward	£3 12. 0

	a Fomentation		4. 0
	an Emetic Powder	Mrs Laycock	0. 6
	three Sudorific Powders		1. 6
	a Mixture		2. 0
	a Lotion for the Eyes	Bartlett's Son	2. 6
25	a Mixture 2/- a Blister	Mrs Maycock	3. 0
	a Mixture 2/- a Bolus	Mrs Noone	2. 6
	a Mixture and paper of Pills	Mary Semple	3. 0
28	the Mixture	Mrs Maycock	2. 0
	pint Mixture	Mrs Smith	4. 0
29	a dose of Pills	Mrs Turner	0. 6
	a Mixture	Mrs Noone	2. 0
	Emetic Powder -/6 Blister 1/-	Master Smith	1. 6
	pint Mixture	Mrs Turner	4. 0
	pint Mixture	Mrs Rodknight	4. 0
31	a dose of Pills -/6 Castor Oil 2/-	extra pauper	2. 6
	a Mixture and Powder	the same pauper	2. 6

	box of Opening Pills	Walker's daughter	1. 0
	Opening Powder	Mrs Turner	1. 0
	box (large) Opening Pills for the use of the House of Industry 2. 0		
	pint Mixture	Smith	4. 0
	box of Pills 1/6 Emetic Powder -/6		2. 0
	box of Opening Pills	Mrs Maycock	1. 6.

Feb

2	a Lotion	Bartlett's Son	2. 0
	a paper of Drops to the eyes repeatedly		0. 0
4	a Bolus, a Mixture and Pills	Mrs James	4. 0
	pint Mixture – box of Pills	Smith	5. 6
		Carried forward	£6 12. 0

	bottle of Drops	Mrs Lace	2. 0
6	a Delivery	Mrs Eydon	10. 6
7	a dose of Pills		0. 6
	a Bolus, a Mixture & Pills	Mrs Lace	4. 0
	attendance during a miscarriage	Mrs Haydon	10. 6
	a Mixture & dose of Pills	Mrs Turner	2. 6
	box of Pills & a Bolus	Mrs Maycock	2. 6
9	a Mixture and Bolus	Mrs Lace	3. 0
	a dose of Pills	Mrs Eydon	0. 6
	a Mixture & three Bolusses	Smith	3. 6
10	a Bolus	Mrs Rodknight	0. 6
	an Opening Bolus	Master Saunders	0. 6
11	a Mixture & dose of Pills	Mrs Turner	2. 6
12	a Mixture & box of Pills	Smith	5. 6
	box of Pills	Mrs Glover	1. 6
13	a Mixture 2/- & a box of Pills	Mrs Bulstrode	3. 6
	two boxes of Pills	Mrs Haycock	3. 0
	a Mixture	Mrs Turner	2. 0
	bottle of Drops – box of Pills	Mrs Lockley	3. 6
15	a dose of Pills	Mrs Turner	0. 6

	a Mixture & box of Pills	Mrs Bicknell	3. 6
16	a Mixture		2. 0
21	box of Pills & twelve Powders	Mrs Turner	3. 6
23	[illegible] 3/6 bottle of Drops & box of Pills		
		Lockley	7. 0
	a Mixture	Mrs McKinch	2. 0
24	a Mixture		2. 0
	8 powders & dose of Pills	extra pauper	3. 6
	three Bolusses & Powders		3. 6
30	bottle of Drops	Master Lockley	2. 0
	a Mixture & box of Pills	extra pauper	4. 0
		Carried forward	£11. 8. 6

March

4	attendance man ulcerated leg		£1. 1. 0
	Plasters – Ointment, Lint & Linseed		0. 0. 0
	three Bolusses	Walker's daughter	1. 6
	box of Pills	Mrs Foster	1. 6
5	a Mixture	Avens	2. 6
7	an absorbed Powder		2. 6
	four Bolusses – Box of Pills	Mrs Foster	1. 6
	an Emetic Powder	J Goode	0. 6
	box of Pills		1. 6
8	box of Pills & Powder	Avens	3. 6
	box of Pills & Emetic Draught	Smith	2. 6
	a Bolus & Emetic Draught	J Goode	1. 6
	two Bolusses	Walter's son	1. 0
	Linseed for Poultice		1. 0
11	pint Mixture & box of Pills	Mrs Foster	5. 6
	Linseed Mixture	Walker's daughter	2. 0
	a Draught – box of Pills & Powder	J Goode	3. 6
14	a Plaster 1/- [illegible] of Hartshorn	Mrs Foster	2. 0
15	Plasters & box of Pills		3. 0
	a Mixture and Electuary	Avens	4. 6
	Opening an abcess in the breast of Walker's daughter		0. 0

	attendance – dressings for the same		10. 6
	box of Pills	J Goode	1. 6
	a Mixture	Avens	2. 0
19	application to the Eyes of [illegible]		1. 6
	Bolus 1/- Salts & Castor Oil		2. 6
	examination of a hernia & truss to Lockley		2. 6
		Carried forward £15. 15. 0	

20	two boxes of Pills (large)	Lockley	4. 0
	Linseed	Avens	1. 0
	box of Pills & Bolus	Rainbow	2. 6
	box of Ointment	Walker's daughter	1. 0
	a Mixture – dose of Pills	Avens	2. 6
21	a Mixture & a Blister	Mrs Rainbow	3. 0
	a pint Mixture & large Plaster	Avens	5. 0
	bottle of Drops	J Goode	2. 0
	box of Ointment	Smith	1. 0
	large box of Bolusses		2. 0
	bottle of Drops and Powders	Mrs Bicknell	4. 6
22	a Mixture & dose of Pills	Mrs Rainbow	3. 0
	box of Pills	Mrs Foster	1. 6
23	a Mixture & Opening Bolus	Mrs Rainbow	3. 0
25	a Mixture & dose of Pills		3. 0
26	a Plaster – box of Pills	J Goode	3. 0
28	a large Blister	Avens	1. 6
29	a pint Mixture		4. 0
	a Mixture	Mrs Rainbow	2. 0
		£18. 4. 6	

Settled H. L. Smith with Mr Marsh
June 24th 1815

COMMENTS:

1] The same names occur regularly – but there were only fifteen residents (including children) in the House of Industry for this period in 1815.

2] All containers (box; bottle; paper etc.) are written in lower case; all medicaments (Drops; Mixtures; Plasters; Leeches etc.) are written with capitals – presumably to denote their importance. I suspect the 'Pills' and 'Mixtures' etc. were of many different varieties, but this would have been of no relevance to the Guardians, and, I suspect, probably closely guarded professional secrets of Henry Lilley Smith.

3] There was no legal requirement (until the 1960s) to label containers of medications with their contents – before then it was infuriating when trying to ascertain what had been swallowed in (say) cases of poisoning/overdose to find the bottle of pills was merely labelled 'The Pills – One to be taken three times daily'.

(b) Itemised account from Dr G Wells to Tredington Overseers (April–December 1834)

To Overseers of the Parish of Tredington

H.G. Wells Surgeon
1834

General Attendance upon the Sick Poor at £13 p. annum from April till Michaelmas   £11. 10. 0

April

| 19 | A lotion Wm Petty | 5. 0 |
| | A pot of ointment | 2. 6 |

May

| 1 | A journey to Upper Quinton | 5. 0 |

	Dressing to leg	2. 6
2	12 leeches for Ed. Scarysbrook	6. 0
4	A journey to Upper Quinton	5. 0
	Dressing to leg	2. 0
6	18 leeches for Ed. Scarysbrook	9. 0
9	A journey to Quinton	5. 0
	Dressing to leg	2. 0
	A Quart mixture	5. 0
11	A piece of plaister	1. 0
15	A journey	5. 0
	Dressing to leg	2. 0
	A Quart mixture	5. 0
27	A journey	5. 0
	A Quart mixture	5. 0
	Dressings to leg	2. 0
28	Plaister	1. 0

June

10	Dressings to leg	2. 6
	Plaister	1. 0
20	Dressings to leg	1. 0

Amount brought forward £15. 14. 0
1834

Sept

22	A Quart lotion	5. 0
	A Quart mixture	5. 0
	A box of pills	2. 0
28	A pot of ointment	2. 0
	A box of pills	2. 6

Oct

5	Dressings to leg	2. 6

	A box of pills	2. 6
	6 powders	2. 6
19	A pot of ointment	2. 6
	A Quart mixture	5. 0
	6 powders	2. 6

Nov

10	A journey to Upper Quinton to Mrs Batchelor	5. 0
16	Dressings to leg	2. 6
	Plaisters	1. 0
	2 rollers	2. 0
20	A journey to Mrs Batchelor	5. 0
	4 powders	1. 6
	A box of pills	2. 6
23	A pot of ointment	2. 6
	Dressings to leg	2. 6
	Lint	1. 0

Dec

7	A pot of ointment	2. 6
	Dressings to leg	2. 6
	Lint	1. 0

Total	£19. 0. 6
(Deduct 3%)	£17. 10. 6

Received from Mr Powers,
Being the amount extra charge
[signed] G Wells 1835

COMMENTS:

1] Dressings for Mrs Batchelor (who appears to have a chronic leg ulcer) are for some reason an 'extra charge' on the annual contract for 'General Attendance upon the Sick Poor'.

2] The price of leeches has fallen dramatically since 1815; perhaps in 1834 they were more widely available and/or easily kept.

3] Dr Wells' reason for the 3% deduction in his fees is not known.

Appendix 3

Dr G Wells, surgeon: correspondence with Overseers, Tredington, relating to his dismissal.

Letter 1

The Overseers Parish of Tredington
1835, G Wells Surgeon

Attendance upon the poor of the Parish of Tredington
from April 2nd to July 28th inclusive at £24 per annum   £7. 15. 3
12 leeches for Harris of Blackwell   6. 0
6 leeches for Plumbe's child, Newbold   3. 0

Total £8. 4. 3

GW will expect from the unhandsome manner in which he has been dismissed by the Overseers of Tredington that this account be discharged immediately: he does not think it worth his while to make any defence for such insignificant charges as are brought against him.

Received the sum of 5 pounds in part payment of the enclosed bill October 31st 1835. G Wells [in a later hand]

Letter 2

Mr Powers
One of the Overseers of the Parish of Tredington

Halford March 8th [1836]

Sir,

I beg to request the immediate settlement of the balance of my account for attending on the sick poor of your Parish from 2nd April to 28th July 1835.

Being on the point of leaving this neighbourhood I cannot wait longer.[73]

Yours etc
G Wells

Acct. delivered £8. 4. 3

Received in part £5. 0. 0

Remaining due £3. 4. 3

Received £2. 0. 0. in discharge of this bill [in a later hand]

---

73   A 'George Wells, surgeon, batchelor aged 31' was married to 'Harriet White, spinster', on 24th May 1838 in Mancetter (near Atherstone, Warwickshire); he was living at the time in Stow-on-the-Wold. Probably one and the same.

Appendix 4

DR AMOS MIDDLETON'S PRESCRIPTION

'I should advise half a pint of the water to be taken first thing in the morning, while the stomach is empty, and the same quantity half an hour after. Should this be found insufficient to keep the bowels open, and to act as a diuretic, then I should recommend a teaspoonful of the salts to be dissolved in a wine glass of the water boiling, and added to each half-pint when taken.

After a full dose, there is generally a slight determination to the head, which is now tested by a sense of drowsiness, and a little fullness across the forehead, but this speedily goes off of itself, or is immediately removed by a walk, ride, or any other gentle exercise; and indeed I should always recommend some exercise after drinking the waters, as it prevents that sense of nausea and apprehension which arises from a quantity of any fluid, when taken into a stomach.'

From *A Chemical Analysis of the Lemington* [sic] *Waters: with a practical dissertation on their medical effects, and instructions for cold and warm bathing' (1814),* by Dr Amos Middleton MD, Physician, Leamington, and consulting physician to the Eye & Ear Infirmary, Southam.

Appendix 5

Conditions treated in the Eye Infirmaries of Southam and Dublin

Conditions treated at the Eye infirmaries of Southam and Dublin (using Southam Infirmary's classification in the 12th Annual Report, 1832):

	Southam (1831–2)	Dublin (1814–17)
Acute inflammation	195	1109
Ditto with thickened eyelids	6	-
Ditto with purulent discharge	7	271[74]
Ditto with pustules of the cornea	7	177
Ditto with ulcers of the cornea	12	282
Ditto of the iris	2	15
Ditto from syphilis[75]	1	11
Ditto from vascular cornea	3	37
Ditto from protrusion of the iris	2	15
Strumous inflammation[76]	14	174
Opacities of the cornea	7	214
Debilities of the retina	41	-

---

74   Incl. 173 children.

75   Surprising there are so few (perhaps because of the high number of children in the total).

76   Inflammation of eyelid margins and eyelashes with damage to the cornea: the term is now obsolete.

Amaurosis[77]	-	33
Paralysis of the eyelids	1	-
Tinea[78]	6	157
Lippitudo[79]	4	96
Excrescences of the conjunctiva	1	25
Inversion of eyelids	4	17
Eversion of eyelids	3	19
Carcinoma (tumour) of eyelids	4	13
Wounds and injuries of the eye	1	273
Diseases of lacrimal passages (tear ducts)	1	523
Cataracts	2	58
Diseases of the ears	28	-
TOTAL	**311**	**2840**

---

77   Probably one and the same as 'debilities of the retina'; both result in partial/total blindness of the eye.

78   A fungal eye infection, often causing damage to the cornea.

79   Inflammation of eyelid margins; 'blepharitis' in today's terminology.

Appendix 6

HUNGERFORD 'LYING-IN' CHARITY – REGULATIONS

'Any woman requiring a "baby box" shall, on receiving a ticket from a Subscriber [thus ensuring she is married, presumably], notify the same, giving (if possible) two months notice, and at the time of her confinement, on sending the ticket to the Subscriber, shall receive an order to a grocer for 1s. worth of soap and grocery and shall receive a "baby box" for her use for one month from the day of her confinement.*

On returning the same in an orderly state she shall receive a gift of clothing for the child (if living) as the funds may allow.**

Six girls selected from Sunday School to be taught plainwork & employed on making up the linen required for the Institution.

Lowest subscription to be 5s. Subscribers of 10s. to be entitled to 3 recommendations, and £1 allows the recommendation of 6 objects in the year.' ***

*

*A 'baby box' contained: two sets of clothing for mother (two shifts; two caps; two petticoats; one long gown; one short gown);

items for the new baby (three infant caps; three shirts; two gowns; twelve nappies) & three sheets; two pillowcases; one counterpane and one testament.

** usually one infant shirt; one cap; one bedgown; one blanket; two nappies.

*** Demeaning for a pregnant woman to be referred to as an 'object', but the context is 'proper object of charity' – the sole criterion of 'eligibility' to receive charity in the Victorian age (as Henry Lilley Smith reminded subscribers to his Infirmary to ensure, when recommending patients for admission).

Appendix 7

CASE REPORT BY HENRY LILLEY SMITH, APRIL 1847

'To the Editor of the *Provincial Medical and Surgical Journal*–

Sir,

The accompanying case occurring at Southam Infirmary appears to me to be of some interest in reference to the physiology of the iris, with which, notwithstanding all that has been done, we are hardly yet sufficiently acquainted. Should you think it likely to gratify your readers, it is much at your service.

I am, Sir,

Yours truly,

Henry Lilley Smith

17 April 1847

A Case of False Pupil

Martha L-------, aged 13, admitted 22nd February 1847.

The Right Eye presents the following appearances:

The pupil is not correctly circular, being as if flattened on its superior margin, but its form to a certain extent varies with the degree of dilatation. The pupil contracts under the influence of light, although more sluggishly than the healthy eye; it expands freely on the application of belladonna.[80]

At the upper part of its ciliary circumference the iris is detached, forming a false pupil, which, when most dilated, is in length about the eighth of an inch, of a fringed irregular form, resembling the opening made when a curtain is partially pulled down. This false pupil varies much in size, being scarcely observable when the natural pupil is dilated, but enlarging when the natural pupil contracts. The false pupil is also, though not to a great extent, affected by the application of belladonna.

When the natural pupil is covered as much as possible and the upper eyelid raised, light can be discerned through the false pupil.

The vision of the right eye is nearly lost, so that she can rarely distinguish the bars of a window, and on being shown a book printed in large type can make out only a number of blank spots. No opacity is discernible in or behind the lens. On using the catoptrical test [forerunner to the ophthalmoscope], the three images are seen. The patient has no pain, ocular spectra [rainbow-coloured lights in the field of vision] or muscae volitantes ['floaters'].

This state is the result of a blow from a stone thrown at her as an infant. She has no useful vision since, and lately the obscurity has, she thinks, increased.

There is no *strabismus convergens* [squint] of the right eye. The left eye is healthy; the iris is of the same colour as that of the right, and the eye being opened or closed produces no effect on the opposite eye.'

---

80   Belladonna = atropine eye drops, from the plant *Atropa belladonna,* or 'Deadly Nightshade', which dilate the pupil, thus allowing better inspection of the eye's interior.

Appendix 8

ANNUAL STATISTICS OF ADMISSIONS TO THE INFIRMARY

Year	Admitted	Cured	Relieved
1818/19	301	136	116
1820	285	111	122
1821	276	147	106
1822	393	254	109
1823	352	225	101
1824	278	115	135
1825	263	140	105
1826	284	170	75
1827	274	184	50
1828	331	190	68
1829	309	176	60
1830	283	168	70
1831	259	184	90
1832	311	193	96
1833	305	187	110
1834	324	210	101

1835	318	234	50
1836	320	240	54
1837	263	210	47
1838	201	196	67
1839	342	209	104
1840	308	217	88
1841	291	205	81
1842	309	240	56
1843	354	321	22
1844	368	317	18
1845	335	312	23
1846	325	309	14
1847	358	300	18
1848	347	199	42
1849	355	206	29
1850	380	308	60
1851	322	277	74
1852	329	343	86
1853	341	250	90
1854	331	270	44
1855	318	250	47
1856	291	256	20
1857	315	261	33

Abbreviations

b.	born
BA	Bachelor of Arts
BMJ	*British Medical Journal*
CRO	County Record Office
CUP	Cambridge University Press
d.	died
FLS	Fellow of the Linnean Society
FRCOphth	Fellow of the Royal College of Ophthalmologists
FRCS	Fellow of the Royal College of Surgeons of England
FRGS	Fellow of the Royal Geographical Society
FSA	Fellow of the Society of Antiquaries
JP	Justice of the Peace
LM	Licentiate in Midwifery (Rotunda Hospital, Dublin)
LRCP	Licentiate of the Royal College of Physicians of England
LRCPI	Licentiate of the Royal College of Physicians in Ireland
LSA	Licentiate of the Society of Apothecaries
MD	Doctor of Medicine
MP	Member of Parliament
MRCP	Member of the Royal College of Physicians of England
MRCPsych	Member of the Royal College of Psychiatrists
MRCS	Member of the Royal College of Surgeons of England
MRCSI	Member of the Royal College of Surgeons in Ireland
OUP	Oxford University Press
Revd	Reverend

Bibliography

BOOKS & JOURNALS

Abel-Smith, Brian *A History of the Nursing Profession* Heinemann, London 1960

Ackroyd, Marcus *et al. Advancing with the Army: Medicine, the Profession and Social Mobility in the British Isles 1790–1850* OUP, Oxford 2007

Albert, Daniel *Men of Vision: Lives of Notable Figures in Ophthalmology* Elsevier, London 1995

Allam, W. *Provident Dispensaries and Friendly Societies Medical Institutions* London 1879

Anderson, John *On Provident Dispensaries; their Object and Their Practical Working* London 1870

Bate, Walter Jackson *John Keats* OUP, Oxford 1966

Bigsby, John *Suggestions Towards the Improvement of the Dispensary at Newark* Newark 1836

Bisset, James *A Descriptive Guide of Leamington Priors* privately printed, Coventry 1814

Brown, Michael *Medicine, Reform and the End of Charity in Early 19C. England* English Historical Review 2006 vol 124 (511): 1353–1388

Burch, Druin *Digging up the Dead: The Life and Times of Astley Cooper, an Extraordinary Surgeon* Chatto & Windus, London 2007

Cave, Lyndon F. *Royal Leamington Spa: Its History and Development* Phillimore, Chichester 1988

Chamberlaine, William *A Dissertation on the Duties of Youths Apprenticed to the Medical Profession* London 1812

Cherry, Steven *Medical Services and the Hospitals in Britain 1860–1939* CUP, Cambridge 1996

Clare, Anthony *Psychiatry in Dissent: Controversial Issues in Thought and Practice* Tavistock Publications, London 1976

Cyriax, R. J. *Nova et Vetera: Henry Lilley Smith MRCS – Founder of Self-supporting Dispensaries* BMJ 18 July 1936

Davidson, Luke *'Identities Ascertained': British Ophthalmology in the First Half of the Nineteenth Century* [SSHM Prize Essay] Soc for the Soc Hist Medicine 1996 Vol 9(3) p313-333

Davis, Celia (ed.) *Rewriting Nursing History* London 1980

Dent, William *Letters to his Mother* National Army Museum 7008/11/2

Digby, Anne *Making a Medical Living: Doctors and Patients in the English Market for Medicine 1720* CUP, Cambridge 1994

Donnison, Jean *Midwives and Medical Men: a History of Inter-Professional Rivalries and Women's Rights* Heinemann, London 1977

Eastoe, Jane *Victorian Pharmacy: Rediscovering Forgotten Remedies and Recipes* Pavilion, London 2010

Editorial, *State of the Sick Poor* London Medical Repository & Review, No. 147 March 1826

Ekirch, Roger A. *Birthright: The true Story that Inspired 'Kidnapped'* Norton, New York 2010

Ellis, Harold *A History of Bladder Stone* Blackwell Scientific Publications, Oxford 1962

Ernst, Waltraud *The role of Work in Psychiatry: Historical Reflections* Indian J Psychiatry 2018 vol60 (2): S248-S252

Fay, C. R. *Life and Labour in the Nineteenth Century* Nonsuch, Stroud 2006

Gordon, William John *The Horse-World of London* London 1893

Gosden, P. H. J. H. *The Friendly Societies of England 1815–1875* Aldershot 1993

Heyward, Paul (Ed.) *Surgeon Henry's Trifles: Events of a Military Life* Chatto & Windus, 1970

Hickinbotham, Peter *The Workhouse Encyclopaedia* History Press, Stroud 2014

Hickinbotham, Peter *Workhouses of the Midlands* Tempus, Stroud 2007

Hindle, Steven *The Birthpangs of Welfare: Poor Relief and Parish Governance in Seventeenth-century Warwickshire* Dugdale Society, Stratford 2000.

Hodgkin, Thomas *On the Mode of Selection and Remuneration of Medical Men for Professional Attendance on the Poor of a Parish or District* Lindfield 1836

Hodgkinson, Ruth *The Origins of the NHS; the Medical Service of the New Poor Law 1834–1871* London Welcome Hist Med library 1967

Holland, P. H. *Self-Providence v Dependence upon Charity: An Essay on Dispensaries* London 1838

Hooper, Robert *Lexicon-Medicum or Medical Dictionary* London 1824

Howard, M. R. *Medical Aspects of Sir John Moore's Corunna Campaign, 1808–1809* J Royal Soc Med 1991 vol 84(5); 299-302

Hunter R. & Macalpine I. *Three Hundred Years of Psychiatry 1535–1860* London 1963

Hull, John *The Philanthropic Repertory of Plans and Suggestions for Improving the Condition of the Labouring Poor* London 1841

Hurry, Jamieson *District Nursing on a Provident Basis* London Scientific Press, 1898

James, R. R. *A History of Ophthalmology in England prior to 1800* Brit J Ophth 1946 30(5): 264-275

Jones, John *Observations on Self-supporting Dispensaries and Suggestions for Rendering Them Generally Efficient* London 1844

Joyce, James *Ulysses* Penguin Classics Penguin Random House, London 2020

Lane, Joan *The Administration of an Eighteenth-Century Warwickshire Parish: Butlers Marston* Dugdale Society, Stratford 1973

Lane, Joan *Social History of Medicine: Health, Healing and Disease in England 1750–1950* Routledge, London 2001

Lane, Joan *Medical Practitioners of Provincial England 1783* Med History 1984 353–371

Lane, Joan *The Provincial Practitioner and his Services to the Poor 1750-1800* Bull Soc Hist Med 1981 28: 10–14

Loftus, Simon *The Invention of Memory: an Irish family Scrapbook, 1560-1934* Daunt Books, London 2013

Loudon, Irvine *Medical Care and the General Practitioner 1750-1850* OUP, Oxford 1986

Loudon, Irvine *Medicine Before the Motor Car* J Royal Soc Med 2009 vol 102(6): 219–222

Loudon, Irvine *Nature of Provincial Medical Practice in 18c England* Med Hist 1985 29: 1–32

Loudon, Irvine *Obstetrics and the General Practitioner* BMJ 1990 vol 301: 703–707

Loudon, Irvine *Origins and Growth of the Dispensary Movement in England* J Bull Hist Med 1981 vol 55 p322–342

Loudon, Irvine *The Origin of the General Practitioner* J Royal Coll Gen Pract 1983 vol 33 p13–18

MacCarthy Fiona *Byron: Life and Legend* John Murray, London 2002

Marryat, Thomas *Therapeutics; or, the Art of Healing* Bristol 1778

Mayerhof, Max *A Short History of Ophthalmia during the Egyptian Campaigns of 1798-1807* Brit J Ophth March 1932 129–152

Medley, Sarah *A Visitor's descriptive guide to Leamington, Warwick and the adjacent towns and villages* Warwick 1826

Middleton, Amos *A Chemical Analysis of the Lemington Waters with a Practical Dissertation on their Medical Effects: and Instructions for Cold and Warm Bathing* Warwick 1814

Nankivell, Charles B. *The Provision of Medical Attendance on the Independent Poor by Provident Dispensaries* BMJ Sept 16th 1871:318–320

Peterkin, Sir Robert *et al.* *Commissioned Officers in the Medical Service of the British Army 1660-1960* Vol 2 Wellcome Hist Med Library 1968

Poole, Benjamin *History of Coventry* Coventry 1852

Priest, W. M. *The Revd Samuel Warneford MA LLD (1763–1855)* BMJ 1969 vol 3: 587-590

Provident Institutions and Hospitals BMJ 27 March 1875 p416–417

Robson, Alastair *'Unrecognised by the World at Large': a Biography of Dr Henry Parsey FRCP* Matador, Kibworth Beauchamp 2017

Rock, Mary *Looking Back at the Sisters' School in Southam* Southam Heritage Collection, Southam 2021

Rose, June *The Perfect Gentleman: The Remarkable Life of Dr James Miranda Barry, the Woman who Served as an Officer in the British Army from 1813 to 1859* London 1977

Rose, Michael E. *The Relief of Poverty 1834–1914* London 1972

Rowley, William *Treatise on the Principal Diseases of the Eye* London 1772

Saunders, John Cunningham *Infirmary for Curing Diseases of the Eye Annual Report* London 1809

Seymour, Richard *Old and New Friendly Societies: a Comparison Between them, with an Account of the Becher and Victoria Clubs recently Established at Stratford-upon-Avon and Alcester* London 1836

Smith, Henry Lilley *Provident Dispensaries; their Social Importance and their Advantages to the Medical Profession* London Medical Journal 1850

Smith, Henry Lilley *Self-Supporting Charitable and Parochial Dispensaries* London 1831

Smith, Henry Lilley *Observations on the Prevailing Practice of Supplying Medical Assistance to the Poor, commonly called the Farming of Parishes* Philanthropic Soc, London 1819

Smith, Henry Lilley *Abstract of a Plan for the Formation of Self-supporting Charitable and Parochial Dispensaries* London 1830

Smith, Henry Lilley *A Classification of Manual Labourers* (Second Annual Report of the Southam Dispensary) Southam 1825

Smith, Henry Lilley *A Diagram to Define the Lives of the Patriarchs* London 1842

Smith, Henry Lilley *Alfred Societies; or a Plan for Very Small Sick Clubs etc.* Southam 1837

Smith, Henry Lilley *Report of a Committee for Conducting an Enquiring into the State of the Sick Poor* Stratford 1827

Smith, Henry Lilley *Second Annual Report of the Southam Dispensary* Southam 1825

Smith, Henry Lilley *Provident Dispensaries: Their Social Importance, and Their Advantages to the Medical Profession* London Journal of Medicine March 1850

Smith, Henry Lilley *Provident or Self-supporting Dispensaries* Assoc Med J 1853 Mar 11; 1 (10): 224

Smith, Henry Lilley *The Society for the Extension of Dispensaries on the Self-supporting Principle Throughout the Kingdom* Report of a Meeting held Warwick 10th July 1858

Smith, William Lilley *Historical Notices and Recollections Relating to the Parish of Southam in the County of Warwickshire Together with the Parochial Registers from AD 1539 and Churchwardens' Accounts AD 1580* 1894 Facsimile Publisher, Delhi, 2015

Smith, William Lilley *Provident Dispensaries* Letter to the BMJ 1 November 1873

Sorsby, Arnold *Defunct Eye Hospitals* Brit J Ophth 1936 Vol 20(2): p77–98

Sorsby, Arnold *Nineteenth Century Provincial Eye Hospitals* Brit J Ophth Sept 1946

Sorsby, Arnold *The Royal Eye Hospital 1857–1957* London 1957

Snow, Stephanie J. *Blessed Days of Anaesthesia: how Anaesthetics Changed the World* OUP, Oxford 2008

Spinks, P. *Stratford-upon-Avon Convalescent Home* Warwickshire History Winter 2005/6 p101–105

Stephens W. B. *Education in Britain 1750–1914* St Martin's Press 1998

Wade, Charles *The History of the Leamington Tennis Court Club 1846–1966* Ronaldson Publications, Oxford 1996

Weir, Neil *History of Medicine: Otorhinolaryngology* Postgrad Med J 2000 Vol 76; 65-69

Wheeler, Simon *Dr Henry Lilley Smith and the Eye and Ear Infirmary* Warwickshire History vol Xlll No 2 winter 2005/6

Wheeler, Simon *Dr Henry Lilley Smith and the Invention of Self-Supporting or Provident Dispensaries* Warwickshire History vol Xlll no 5 summer 2007

Whitfield, Michael *The Dispensaries; Healthcare for the Poor Before the NHS* Authorhouse UK, Milton Keynes 2016

Wildman, Stuart *'He's only a Pauper whom Nobody owns': Caring for the Sick in the Warwickshire Poor Law Unions, 1834–1916* Dugdale Society, Stratford 2016

Wilde, Sir William *Practical Observations on Aural Surgery and the Nature and Treatment of Diseases of the Ear* Fannin & Co., Dublin 1853

Williams, Samantha *Practitioners' Income and Provision for the Poor: Parish Doctors in the Late Eighteenth and Early Nineteenth Centuries* Social History of Medicine Vol 18; issue 2, Aug 2005 p159–186.

Wilmot, John *Advice and Medicine for the Working Classes: the Leamington and Warwick Provident Dispensaries 1869–1913* Warwickshire History Vol XVI no 1 Summer 2014

Wilson, Alyson & Fry, Claire *Clapham Through Time* Amberley Publishing, Stroud 2015

Woodward, John *To Do The Sick No Harm: a Study of the British Voluntary Hospital System to 1875* Routledge, London 1974

Woodford, Leonard *A Medical Student's Career in the Early Nineteenth Century* Medical History vol XIV No.1 January 1970

Woodford, L. W. *A Young Surgeon in Wellington's Army* Old Woking Unwin Bros 1976

Yeatman, John C. *Remarks on the Medical Care of the Parochial Poor* Longmans, London 1818

Yeatman, John C. *Remarks on the Necessity for Parliamentary Interference Respecting the Medical Care of Sick and Hurt*

Paupers Letter to *The Lancet* 13 July 1833

Young, A. *A Six Weeks Tour through the Southern Counties of England & Wales* London 1768

THESES & DISSERTATIONS

Bogle, Richard *From Charity to Providence: Influences on the Organisation of Dispensaries in the Early 19th Century* Dissertation for the Diploma in the History of Medicine (DHMSA), Society of Apothecaries of London 2012

Burnby, Juanita *A Study of the English Apothecaries from 1660–1760* PhD thesis, University of London 1979

Denny, Elaine *The Emergence of the Occupation of District Nurse in 19c. England* PhD thesis, University of Nottingham 1999

House, Carolanne Margaret *The Development of Rural District Nursing in Gloucestershire 1880–1925* PhD thesis, University of Gloucestershire 2004

Negrine, Angela *Medicine and Poverty: a Study of the Poor Law Medical Services of the Leicester Union 1867–1914* PhD thesis, University of Leicester 2008

Pinches, Sylvia *Charities in Warwickshire in 18c. & 19c.* PhD thesis, University of Leicester 2000

Ritch, Alistair *Medical Care in the Workhouses in Birmingham and Wolverhampton 1834–1914* PhD thesis, University of Birmingham 2015

Wheeler, Simon *Henry Lilley Smith (1788–1859): Surgeon, Philanthropist and Originator of Provident Dispensaries* MA thesis, University of Warwick 1996

Wildman, Stuart *Local Nursing Associations in an Age of Nursing Reform 1860–1900* PhD Thesis, University of Birmingham 2012

Williams, Richard Sylvanus *A Survey of Staffordshire Medical Practitioners in 1851*

(draft paper) University of Exeter 2018

WEBSITES

British Medical Journal
The Lancet
Provincial Medical & Surgical Journal
The London Medical Gazette
General Medical Register

Coventry Provident Dispensary Annual Reports
Commissioners in Lunacy Ninth Report 1856

Kelly's Directory 1872
Pigot & Co. *National Commercial Directory* 1828–1829
Leamington Society *A Walk Around Royal Leamington Spa* 1962
    (revised 1981)

via britishnewspaperarchive.com
    Leamington Spa Courier
    Northampton Mercury
    Coventry Herald
    Birmingham Gazette

bmsgh.org (midland-ancestors.uk) *Birmingham and Midlands Society for Genealogy & Heraldry*
british-history.ac.uk *A History of the County of Warwick; Southam* Vol 6 p219–226
british-history.ac.uk *A History of the County of Warwick; Coventry The Provident Dispensary, Bayley Lane* Vol 8 p275–298
districtadvertisers.co.uk *Remembering the Warneford* (by Irene Cardall)
historicengland.org.uk *Former Clapham General Dispensary*
leamingtonhistory.co.uk *Forgotten local history: the Leamington Provident Dispensary*
londonlives.org *London Lives 1690–1800: Parish Relief*

nhshistory.net *Development of the London Hospital System 1823– 2015*

ourwarwickshire.org.uk *Nineteenth Century Allotments in Southam* (by Anne Langley)

ourwarwickshire.org.uk *Lady Amherst's Earache* (by Beck Hemsley)

rcpe.ac.uk *Medical treatment for the poor; The Dispensary*

rcophth.ac.uk *Short History of Ophthalmology*

richardjohnbr.blogspot.com *Looking at History: A horse-drawn Society?*

rnib.org.uk *Blindness in the 18th century*

workhouses.org.uk *Poor Law and Workhouse Administration and Staff*

workhouses.org.uk *Southam, Warwickshire*

Index

HLS = Henry Lilley Smith